Advance Praise

"Karen Lorre's love radiates to you as you read *Chronic Pleasure*. You can trust that Karen is the real deal – she embodies *Chronic Pleasure* and teaches you to do the same."

– Deepak Chopra

"When I first met Karen Lorre a decade ago, she was physically and emotionally weakened by years of stress. Today, Karen is profoundly physically younger and super vibrant, illuminated with passion and loving radiance. Karen's amazing life transformation reminds me of the classic scene in the movie *When Harry Met Sally,* where Meg Ryan, in a diner, pretends to have an orgasm. One of the observing diners turns to a waitress and says, 'I'll have what she is having!'

"In *Chronic Pleasure*, Karen reveals her path to enlightenment through reprogramming her consciousness, and in the process, evolved from victim to master of her life. While her story may sound 'new-agey,' it is all scientifically based. A fundamental principle of quantum physics, the most tested and validated of all the sciences, acknowledges as fact that consciousness is creating our life experiences. While a conscious knowledge of quantum physics principles is profound, it is only through the practice of engaging those principles that we can truly experience their power.

"Chronic Pleasure provides a life changing compilation of personal and client experiences that reveal how thoughts, emotions, and actions shape every aspect of our perceived reality. More importantly, this book provides a treasury of hands-on practices where Karen's words can be turned into positive life-changing actions. Her vision, outlook and intentions in creating a happier and healthier world are an inspiration and a practice for manifesting self-empowerment. For an antidote to the pain of today's world of personal and global chaos, read Karen Lorre's *Chronic Pleasure."*

- Bruce H. Lipton, Ph.D.,
Cell biologist and author of the bestselling *The Biology of Belief,*
Spontaneous Evolution (with Steve Bhaerman)
and *The Honeymoon Effect*

"Bravo! In *Chronic Pleasure,* Karen Lorre's deep and joyous commitment to truly unconditional love shines through on every page. So few books on the Law of Attraction let us know that it can be fun! Karen is spot-on in reminding us that the solution to misery isn't 'less misery.' It's MORE JOY!"

– Gay Hendricks, Ph.D.
Bestselling author of *The Big Leap* and *Conscious Loving*

"Chronic Pleasure is a rapturous read, to be experienced on multidimensional levels of Being. Read with an open heart-soul-mind-body and allow yourself to be guided on a rippling, resonant pleasure journey. This book is a gift, imbued with Karen Lorre's expansive, open heart. Imminently practical with astonishing real-life tales of transformation, *Chronic Pleasure* is a divinely organized Re-Source for application in one's life Now."

– Jennifer Mason

"An original approach to the physical, emotional, and spiritual problems that plague the modern human being. The healing power Karen has developed jumps right off the page. Best of all, she shares it with the reader in a simple but inspiring way. A book you don't just read – you feel."

– Phil Stutz
Co-author of *The Tools*

"Who can write a book called *Chronic Pleasure*? Karen Lorre can. Her positivity is nuclear. She shines bright as the stars in the heavens."

– Chris Carter
Creator of *The X-Files*

"I've known Karen for a long time, and the transformation I've seen her go through is nothing short of miraculous! From being on the brink of giving up on healing her body and heart, Karen found a path of self-love, massive divine connection, and authentic expression that healed her whole life and opened up her capacity for healing others in a deep and profound way – and for the first time she's put everything into her book, *Chronic Pleasure*. With all the self-help books that offer nothing new, it's so exciting to see someone come along and take everything to the next level! Karen is the real deal, a true master, and one of the most loving, caring, generous souls I know. Read this book, put it into practice, soak in the field of her consciousness – and watch lifelong issues heal and a life of true joy and passion emerge!"

– Derek Rydall
Bestselling author of *Emergence* and *The Abundance Project*
www.DerekRydall.com

"Genius! Most books on the Law of Attraction merely pay lip service to the idea that our feelings are the key to getting what we want. In *Chronic Pleasure*, Karen Lorre offers us a clear, step-by-step guide to rousing the intense, positive emotions that help us transform our bodies and our lives. Even better, she manages to do this by genuinely embodying what she's teaching: Karen's irrepressible joy, wonder, and lust for life are palpable in every single sentence, and instantly ignite these same feelings in us as we read. Bravo!"

– Marc Rosenbush

Co-Founder of SuperMind Apps and Creator/Executive Producer of *Conversations with Neale* and *Conscious Love Stories* (Amazon Prime)

"This book is a beautiful reminder of how powerful our mind and brain can be in our lives and how we can control more than we think we can in our own lives through meditation and finding positivity in our lives. Karen has beautifully written this book in a narrative style that is easy to read and is interspersed with some amazing poems that she has written. Having met Karen and having experienced her love and positivity, I can say that she has not only transformed herself but continues to pass on that love and advice to others. Would definitely recommend this book, especially for those seeking to find ways to transform themselves and find more love and pleasure in their lives."

– Anu Acharya
CEO, Mapmygenome

"Every teacher has some beautiful and unique perspective and gift. But, after interviewing hundreds of the most amazing thought leaders in the self-help and spiritual world and meeting spectacular people from all over the world I have to say, publicly, that Karen is at a whole new level of teacher . . . and, more importantly, at a whole new level of human being! And you can feel it on every page of this book."

– Richard Greene
Author, Journalist, Lawyer, Communication Strategist
and Motivational Speaker
www.RichardGreene.org

"I just finished *Chronic Pleasure* and WOW, it was *so* good! I literally loved every word. Even on my first read-through I felt all Karen's love *really* come through and I was *so* lifted up. As I read, my joy just rose and rose and rose. I am now more committed than ever to connect with who I really am as I reach new levels of love and healing. And the book is not only inspirational, it is highly practical. Karen Lorre shares how high-on-life she is, but she also lays out an effective (and really fun) path to follow to get there. I am looking forward to going back through the book (many, many times) and trying the suggested practices. I've read hundreds of books about the Law of Attraction (I'm a coach too) and *Chronic Pleasure* is different; it suggests some fabulous practices that are truly unique, that can take our spirits and bodies to a whole new level. I love Karen Lorre. I love *Chronic Pleasure*, I love me, *and* I thank Karen for sharing her stories, her inspirations, her successes, her humor, her passion, her truth, and her pleasure with us. This book is going to rock the universe! I am still buzzing from it! Karen Lorre is a wonder."

– Su Crutchfield

"I was eager to read the book written by Karen because I listened to her yummy meditations and every time I did so it made me feel stable and resistant to stress. I wondered how she became so loving and positive. As a mum of two kids I often feel hardship and overwhelm. Reading this book changed my view on life completely. I feel indefinitely loved and supported. The book is short and easy to read. It contains advice on how to create bliss out of all areas of your life. It is so empowering and inspirational. When I read the story how Karen felt before finding her way to experience constant pleasure (I could relate in many things) and how she feels now it made me cry. Blissful life, health, and happiness are available to everyone!

"I wrote down so many things from the book. I feel awesome just thinking about practising them. Many of the things Karen talks about in the book are well known or heard of, but the way she is interpreting them, using them, combining them is genius and effective. I feel much more loving and practising compassionate thoughts towards my children makes it easy for me to stay calm and connected to them. I noticed that my teen son, in a few days of practising pleasure exercises, opened up several times to me about what he feels and thinks. He did it only rarely before. He even asked me to call him more often with nice names like sweetheart, sunshine, darling. Big surprise!

"This pleasurable softness slowly fills in my house and I am so grateful I was fortunate enough to access so much wisdom and knowledge from this book."

– Margarita Vid

"Karen Lorre captures (as best one can) her energetic, high spirited, compassionate, and insightful nature, and transcribes it into her bestselling book, *Chronic Pleasure*. Those who have had the delightful pleasure of knowing her as friend, colleague, or client – as well as those who have not yet had this lovely experience – can benefit now and forever from her enthusiastic, playful wisdom expressed in these pages. One can either climb a tall mountain in India in search of a guru, search out Southern France for a monk, figure out where in China the Shaolin priests reside – or more easily, just read (and participate in the many exercises of) Karen's book! If a guru is defined (in Joel Mlerko's words) as 'a counselor, who helps mold values, shares experiential knowledge as much as literal knowledge, an exemplar in life, an inspirational source and who helps in the spiritual evolution of a student', Karen is surely one!

"She mixes her own brand of how to feel good into the melting pot of Hicks, Lipton, Dispenza, and Chopra. She sprinkles these with her own seasoned knowledge gained through her personal, unique experiences which she shares with us so freely. One can swear there is also, in this opus, a taste of Csikszentmihályi, Maslow, and the Tao. Whatever the sources, Karen serves her dish in delicious spoonfuls meant to be digested one at a time, but culminating in a soul-satiating blend of practices that lift one to unimaginable heights. If this whets your appetite, dig in! It's a bountiful feast!"

– Neal Stolar, MD-PhD

"I was titillated while reading the book *Chronic Pleasure* by Karen Lorre. I've always believed that people know the truth when they hear it and I felt the divine truth in words throughout the book.

There are many masters on the planet that have evolved into gurus of sorts. What Karen Lorre expresses in this book are the practice steps that create masters. We are all powerful beings of love. This book shows the path in processes that lead to a happy, fun, pleasurable, and exciting life. It takes the momentum of practice to create the energy to make it happen. This book gives the reader some amazing tools along with real life examples to manifest fun and pleasure.

"I am in a texting mastermind positive word game with Karen and Norma Eckroate. We have taken turns with positive words every single day for over four years. I've known Karen Lorre for many more years and can testify she is the example of chronic pleasure.

I'm so excited to have my clients read this book."

– Carilyn Davidson
Author of C Davidson Tax and Mastermind Word Game Buddy

"Karen Lorre has written an inspiring and delightful book. It contains remarkable insights, pragmatic advice, and spiritual wisdom; all for helping the reader to lead a full and rewarding life. To get the most out of the book, the reader should follow the author's advice and read with a notepad handy to write down those "ah-ha" moments that the book inspires. As she mentions early on in the book, each reader will have their own unique interpretation and insights in reaction to the book. And it is through those insights that the book becomes most helpful. In the end, this book is about you, the reader.

"To me, this book is essentially about prayer. One of my first 'ah-ha' moments was when she states that every thought, emotion, and action is a prayer. This is the same idea as prayer without ceasing that has been promoted by Christian mystics through the ages. Only she makes clear that one is not engaging in a mental prayer while thinking, feeling, and acting; but that the thoughts, emotions, and actions *are* the prayer; and that distinction is critical if one is to feel the beneficent reciprocity from the Universe, from God.

"The practice of heartfull meditation, which is central to the book, can be life transforming. Another 'ah-ha' moment occurred when Karen explained how our brains interpret signals from the heart. When we are heart-centered we can open up and receive the bounty from the Universe. She is saying that meditation and prayer should be heartfull as opposed to mindful; similar to religious centering prayer. After all, Catholics for ages have prayed to the Immaculate Heart of Mary, not the immaculate brain!

"I was profoundly touched when the author discussed the sexual trauma that she suffered as a child. How she has managed to overcome it is truly inspiring. She has even been in contact with her abuser's spouse, and was able to express love and forgiveness. What she explains is that learning to embrace and love your fate will allow the pain to transform you into the beautiful person that you are. Karen Lorre is a beautiful person, and so are you, so are all of us; that is her ultimate message in this book. I'm thankful that Karen had the heartfull strength to share that part of her life and her triumph over it.

"Karen Lorre lives her life as a goddess and calls upon the reader to do the same. I'm reminded of the words of Meister Eckhart, a thirteenth century Christian mystic; 'God gives birth to the Son as you, as me, as each one of us. As many beings, as many gods in God.' I thank her for writing a book that helps one to become a god in God, and I love her for that."

– Stephen Lobb

"I absolutely adore Karen's book. I have listened to Abraham-Hicks for over twenty years and this was the boost that I personally needed to get into my vortex and stay here. INFINITE YAY!!!!! In my opinion, this book will most certainly give you the means to lift yourself up into more expanded feelings of joy and happiness, into the frequency of your desires, when you do the practices. Do it just for the fun of it, as Karen says. And not only is it super fun, but Karen makes it super easy too. With her help, it truly is child's play. I highly recommend this book if you enjoy doing inner work."

— Eva Wu

"*Chronic Pleasure* is a pure gem just as is the author, Karen Lorre. Reading it has already changed my life!

"I feel so exhilarated, loved, worthy, and more connected with each of the practices suggested.

"It simply clarified principles that I already knew, and made them so practical and easy to apply. Karen's chronic pleasure is contagious!

I am appreciating the contrast that life brings me, seeing it as an opportunity to live the new challenges, by playing with the practices in her book. I'm glad for the opportunity for expansion, to feel more joy, more unconditional love, more everything wonderful...

"I feel so much energy and love for myself, and for all."

— Rima Nasreddine

"In her book, *Chronic Pleasure*, Karen Lorre shares her personal journey and the wisdom that she has diligently optimized over many years to unfold a life that is overflowing with pleasure. She has followed the path of Master teachers, who have told us for millennia that 'It is done unto you as you believe.' Karen brings clarity to the beliefs and practices that keep us stuck in the old paradigms of lack and limitation and gives us numerous examples of how to crack the code of Law of Attraction. She also presents forty-three easy-to-follow and powerful 'practices' to magnify and optimize our potential. I believe we are on this planet to learn how powerful we really are as loving spiritual beings. Karen's roadmap to chronic pleasure is a magnificent path to access our divinity. It is a true blessing to us all that she is sharing her wisdom with us."

– Norma Eckroate

Author of *The Medical Marijuana Handbook*; coauthor of *The Natural Cat*, *The Dog Whisperer*, and *The Puppy Whisperer*, among others

"OMG I love reading this book! I'm looking forward to starting over again and doing the fun exercises. But I have to say that I had the experience of extreme pleasure and joy while reading the pages. It's as if I could feel the divine source through Karen to me directly from the screen into my heart, soul, body. I feel so much more open to receive and to give right now. During this short time I miraculously lost ten pounds I've been struggling with for years to lose. That's crazy!!"

– Bettina Skye

Chronic Pleasure

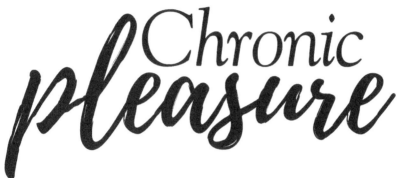

Chronic pleasure

Use the Law of Attraction to
Transform Fatigue and Pain
into Vibrant Energy

Karen Lorre

NEW YORK

LONDON • NASHVILLE • MELBOURNE • VANCOUVER

Chronic Pleasure

Use the Law of Attraction to Transform Fatigue and Pain into Vibrant Energy

© 2020 Karen Lorre

Published in New York, New York, by Morgan James Publishing in partnership with Difference Press. Morgan James is a trademark of Morgan James, LLC. www.MorganJamesPublishing.com

ISBN 9781642795110 paperback
ISBN 9781642795127 eBook
ISBN 9781642796100 audioBook
Library of Congress Control Number: 2019902360

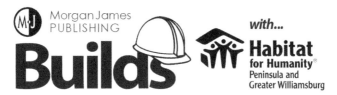

Morgan James is a proud partner of Habitat for Humanity Peninsula and Greater Williamsburg. Partners in building since 2006.

Get involved today! Visit
MorganJamesPublishing.com/giving-back

This book is dedicated to all the people in this world who want to feel better physically or emotionally. I feel epic love for you. I feel my greatest happiness is contributing to your happiness and well-being.
Thank you.

Table of Contents

BlissClaimer
(AKA: Disclaimer!)

This book represents my lifelong study, my heart, my spirit, and my deep desire to share the experiences and perspectives that I believe can bring joy, comfort, and love to those who read it and do the practices in this book.

It was, however, not written by a medical professional, is not medical advice, and is not intended to replace medical advice or treatment from licensed medical practitioners.

Please enjoy this book, but also consult with trusted medical practitioners for any mental, emotional, or physical challenges you might be experiencing.

You reading this book is an acknowledgement that you take full responsibility for yourself and your well-being.

With love, Karen.

Introduction

Why I Wrote This Book for You

I feel so much love for you. This book is a love letter to you because I want you to feel the epic chronic pleasure I feel.

I feel so blessed. I used to go to a therapist and lots of doctors. I went every week to therapy, and I felt sicker both physically and mentally.

I felt hopeless. I wanted to die, just to get some relief. I felt chronic pain, I was falling asleep sometimes fifteen times a day, all my relationships were ruined. I felt so despairing.

Then, I found the Law of Attraction…

I already had a good understanding of neuroscience, epigenetics, psychobiology, how to induct myself and others into a deep state of relaxation and I had a mysterious (to me at the time) ability to channel Source Energy. When I understood the Law of Attraction, I felt the clarity of how to heal my body.

Whether you know all of these things or not does not really matter. What matters is that if you read this book and follow the practices, you will experience massive benefits. I will share more about that soon.

I created a meditation for myself to listen to daily, and I also downloaded from the Universe several practices that I did daily, which I will share with you. My body and I transformed within a few months of listening to that meditation and doing the various practices. My meditations and practices healed things that doctors had been trying to heal for years.

My meditations and practices for my body transformed my body from a state of chronic pain, no energy, narcolepsy, depleted adrenals, hair loss, weak nails, thinning eyebrows, anemia, thyroid issues, needing glasses, and osteopenia, to chronic pleasure, which feels like I am being massaged on the inside of my body any time I want. I feel the energy in my body rushing up from my feet to my head and beyond in a way that feels like a sweeping inner caress. I feel incredible contractions and pulsing in my sex organs that sends energy up my body and feels erotic. I feel my heart filled with pure, shining love. Food tastes incredible. Drinking water feels so luxurious. I could go on and on!

I also feel my energy increasing daily. I feel incredible, vibrant energy – I often feel like a little kid with my energy (even though I don't even drink caffeine or any stimulant). I feel so excited to skip and cartwheel and play. I feel my adrenals relaxed and healthy. My thyroid feels perfectly balanced naturally now with no drugs.

This boundless natural energy during the day now feels like the narcolepsy is gone. My bones feel soooo strong naturally (the doctor was amazed). I have great iron levels in my blood naturally now. My hair has grown back thicker and healthier, my eyesight has improved and is continuing to improve. I can read things now that I could not read without glasses twenty years ago. Now it feels easy to read them!

This all transformed in my body within a few months of listening to the meditations I made for myself and doing the practices I discovered. My friends and family were amazed.

Everything I wanted began to flow in with such consistency and ease. My life felt easier and easier... I felt richer and healthier and clearer and happier each time I listened to a meditation I made, and each time I did one of these practices.

I fired my therapist (even thought I still love and appreciate him!) I fired my doctors. (Except for one doctor but that's because he's my friend!)

My therapist couldn't believe how I transformed so easily, both physically and emotionally and energy-wise. My doctors were shocked.

That is why I am writing this book.

I feel so much love for you, and for me, and I want you to feel as good as you can too. I want you to feel the release of emotional or physical pain and fatigue so you can feel the incredible chronic pleasure I have and the incredible energy and all the goodness I have and more. I want you to feel like you are being massaged on the inside, like your heart feels wide open and filled with love. I want you to feel your body energized, feeling like you want to skip and dance and play. I feel so confident this book will benefit you, because my clarity transformed my body and my life so easily and so quickly and these practices have worked for many hundreds of my clients.

Now, I feel so thankful to say that people come to me and they get what they want, usually within nine sessions with me.

Sometimes people want more sessions, because they say I am so much fun to play with, but everyone always gets a ton of that which they were seeking in the *first* nine sessions with me. This book will feel like you are getting your own private session with me whenever you want. The practices in this book will nourish you any time you do them.

Of course, there are benefits to having one-on-one or group coaching as well – in one-on-one or group sessions I can help with specific issues and help you to remove unconscious blocks (which is not within the scope of this book), but even without any coaching sessions, you will find your ability to feel more and more pleasure and more and more energy increasing each time you do any of these practices.

It feels like such a beautiful honor to be a benefit and to have easy, effortless solutions for every situation that I or others have encountered so far. I have channeled many hundreds of these meditations and shared my practices now with many hundreds of clients and the consistency of my clients loving sessions with me and raving about them to me feels so very gratifying! It feels obvious I have found a path that is effective and powerful because I am consistently told that I strike the right vibrational chord in everyone I work with – clients tell me that over and over and over. I feel honored to share all I can with you in this book, so you, too, will experience all these benefits.

I feel very thankful that I was inspired to offer my coaching and meditations to others, and that from the very first day I offered them, I got my first clients.

I feel thankful that I have been booked almost every day since then – unless I book out for time to do other things. It all feels like effortless abundance. And I feel thrilled that I am distilling the practices I created and discovered into this book and into online classes that will enable you to release all physical and emotional pain and fatigue and to have all the pleasure and energy you want.

I love you!

Karen Lorre

Chapter 1:

Use the Law of Attraction to Heal Your Emotional or Physical Fatigue and Pain

D o you know the Law of Attraction, but still have emotional or physical pain or fatigue?

I imagine you have wanted to feel healthy and energized for a long time. Maybe you have tried many different options. Maybe some have helped, but not fully.

Maybe you understand the Law of Attraction, but you feel your understanding does not sink into your body enough. That is okay. Does your understanding feel more intellectual or mental, instead of it being a deep visceral KNOWING? Are you wanting to get your emotions and body to be impacted in a positive way?

Do you try to figure out what you are doing wrong that is keeping this issue present?

Do you get upset with yourself when you are not feeling good?

Does your mind get overwhelmed and you need time to process things?

Do you often hesitate to make plans because you are not sure how you will feel? Have your work life or relationships suffered because of your pain or fatigue?

Have doctors told you that they don't know what is wrong?

Or worse, have they told you that you may never recover?

You are not alone. What you are experiencing is totally understandable. You are not wrong for what you are experiencing. You are about to step into the solution with your body, mind, and spirit. You want to feel good. I feel certain you have tried so many things. You have probably sought out so many solutions.

Maybe you go up and down in energy throughout the day. Maybe you get triggered and then have an endless loop of beating yourself up. Maybe you have lived with pain for a very long time and it feels impossible to shift. Perhaps you have said or done things in your pain or fatigue that have hurt your relationships. Perhaps your work feels too challenging right now.

It does not feel good to not feel good. I feel such gentle compassion for you. Perhaps your whole-body aches. Do you just feel so tired that you almost want to give up? Maybe it does not feel safe to drive. Maybe you feel so tired in social situations. Maybe you feel scared you will fall asleep or not be fully present in social situations.

And yet, within you, you *know* that you are meant to feel good and to have the energy and ability to do what you want to do, to be what you want to be, and to have what you want to have. This is all how I used to feel. That's why I know you can feel so much better too!

What is the Law of Attraction?

Many people understand the Law of Attraction, but they are still not getting the things they desire.

To me, it is the way the Universe listens to *everything* we think, feel, and say. The Universe's response to us is a perfect match to the essence of all that we think, feel, and say. There is no time that the Law of Attraction is not operating. In every moment, we are creating our lives. We create our lives in the car, in the shower, in our conversations with our kids, partners, friends parents, or coworkers, etc.

The Law of Attraction is also very individual. What I mean is that even if the rest of the world believes something negative, if I am believing something that feels nourishing to my being, then I will never have negative experiences even if that is what everyone else is experiencing, or if I do experience something unwanted it won't have a lasting negative effect upon me and it will turn into a huge gift.

Here is another way to look at the Law of Attraction:

Imagine that you are buying experiences and things with only your emotions...but you can only buy what is equal to your emotion.

So if you are wanting something full of love, you would have to be feeling full of love to buy it.

If you happen to feel afraid, you could only buy things that will scare you more.

If you want to buy something rich, you would have to be feeling abundant and rich to buy it...

That is actually how this world works. We are exchanging our emotions for experiences or things that match them.

If you want better experiences or things, it feels fun to start practicing feeling better emotions.

The Law of Attraction is all about me (and you) taking *full* responsibility for everything we are living, knowing that we created it.

But don't let that scare you. Even if you have been living something less than what you want or something really terrible, you can switch it around much more quickly than you may think. The Law of Attraction does not care about what you focused on yesterday. It only cares what you are focusing on now. And since the Law of Attraction is in action in every moment, this book looks at common places where most people are unaware of their negative beliefs and shows you ways to shift them. I feel masterful at using the Law of Attraction for my benefit and you will feel masterful too, after reading this book.

You can use a clear understanding of the Law of Attraction to heal your emotional or physical pain and fatigue. That is what I have done and what I have taught many of my private clients and those in my workshops. You can trust that I know the process.

I feel clear that pain and excess fatigue are not necessary, and I feel so much love for you, which is why I wrote this book.

Where you are is okay, don't worry. I feel confident you can feel all the health and well-being in your body that you want.

It's taken me a long time to learn the things I will share with you. I had been dealing with pain and fatigue for my whole adult life and even when I learned the Law of Attraction, it took me years to really find the secrets that keep me in wonderful, thriving health, vibrant energy, and chronic pleasure. These secrets that really worked came through great insights that I then put into daily practice. I created a path for myself that transformed my whole body and my whole life. This is what I feel so thrilled to share with you.

Focusing on your body's health is important, but there is so much more to health than that. It feels so strange to know that many people are contributing to their pain and fatigue with simple beliefs they acquired from school, parents, the news, culture, and so many other places. We will unlock many of those together.

The body is a complex and extraordinary thing. It is actually so brilliant that it is still not understood fully by science. And yet, the body is also very responsive when you know how to work with it. In fact, your body *wants* you to work with it in the ways I will show you. Your body will thank you over and over if you continue reading this book and if you follow the practices I suggest.

For a lot of people, making the time to be healthy does not feel like a priority. There are work, children, and responsibilities to focus upon, and while all of that is totally understandable and important, when you feel wonderful in your body, when you have no physical or emotional pain and you feel energized, when you feel actual pleasure in your body, you are going to be a better parent, a better friend, a better worker, a better spouse… in fact, as you read this book and do the practices, you will find all areas of your life improving as your body improves as well. When you use the tools in this book, you will find an abundance of time that has been hidden behind your stress and worry.

If you don't know the complex genius mechanics of your body, that's okay. You are right on track. I have found recovery and wonderful health while understanding only what I needed to understand.

I am writing this book because I have let go of all my pain, both physical and emotional, and I feel so much exquisite pleasure and abundant energy. I am able to process and learn things so much quicker and easier than I ever could before. I am writing this book because I feel incredible love for you, so I am sharing everything I can that will help you feel wonderful in your body and mind.

But it's up to you.

I will share everything I know that helped my emotions and body and the emotions and bodies of my clients. And even though reading this book is important, what's most important is the action part that will cause you to feel incredible as you do it. You will find such massive benefits from doing the practices – even if they don't seem to make sense and seem to have nothing to do with what your body is experiencing.

If you commit to really reading this book to the end and to taking each practice as I suggest them, you will feel so much better and you will either experience the freedom you were born to feel or have a clear plan to follow to experience it more and more each day that you practice it.

You were born to feel healthy and to have pleasure in your body. You were born to have abundant energy. You were born to be able to do, be, and have all that you desire.

You are about to step into a magical pathway that will provide you with what you were born to live.

I know that what I am suggesting works because it has literally transformed my body and my entire life and the lives and bodies of many of my clients.

The best way to read this book is to read it through, get the understanding, and then go back and do the practices one by one. And then keep doing the practices because they do feel wonderful to do!

Get a journal or use your phone or computer and take notes and do the practices there. It'd feel even better and more helpful if you take what I suggest and make it your own, so it makes total sense to you.

Everyone is different and this book can be used to address your specific needs and desires regarding healing your pain, fatigue, and more. You will find great relief and more benefits in every area of your life than you ever imagined by doing these practices. You will find yourself having "aha" moment after "aha" moment. Write these new insights down someplace where you can keep them. I have a page in my phone under the notes section where I write down my "aha"s. You can do it in your way. These new insights will source you and guide you in ways that will surprise and delight you.

As you move through this book and as you live your life, you will find more and more ways to apply the practices suggested here. Each time you do these practices you will feel better and better – if you do them in the right way – which I will discuss in a little bit. There are two ways you can do the practices: one way can benefit you and one way can harm you. I will guide you to use only the way that can benefit you!

It's valuable that you realize that this wisdom took me years to experiment with, to distill, and to test on others, finding that it worked for them, too.

So, if you are reading this book just once it will not sink in and do the magic that it has the power to do. I suggest you keep this book someplace where you like to read and refer to it often. I suggest you read it any time you have a new challenge coming up that you don't know how to deal with. Let yourself become saturated in the love and wisdom that is here. Let this book and these practices drench you in more clarity than you have ever had.

I wish I could just wave a magic wand and let you have the perfect emotions and body the way you want (I am working on that!! Giggle!). But this all depends upon you and your willingness to do these practices in a consistent way and in the way that benefits you and to reap the benefits.

I wrote this book feeling so full of love and pleasure and I feel curious if you can feel that as you read!

Commitment:

As mountaineer William Hutchison Murray said so wonderfully, "Until one is committed, there is hesitancy, the chance to draw back, always ineffectiveness. Concerning all acts of initiative (and creation), there is one elementary truth, the ignorance of which kills countless ideas and splendid plans: that the moment one definitely commits oneself, then Providence moves too. All sorts of things occur to help one that would never otherwise have occurred. A whole stream of events issues from the decision, raising in one's favor all manner of unforeseen incidents and meetings and material assistance, which no man could have dreamt would have come his way. I have learned a deep respect for one of Goethe's couplets:

Whatever you can do, or dream you can, begin it.
Boldness has genius, power, and magic in it!"

I have loved that quote all my life and it has fueled me so many times when I wanted to quit.

That commitment is what I invite you to have. A commitment to yourself. A commitment to healing your body. A commitment to having fun and to your alignment. A commitment to living in the solution. A commitment to reading this book to the end, doing the practices, and finding all the gifts – and reading this book again whenever you need help. When you do that, you will find every area of your life benefits.

The way I have healed is different than what others teach and so when I teach it, either with a one-on-one client, in groups or in workshops, it's something unique, and here's how.

First, I don't just deal with your body. I know that everything is connected, so I teach you how to transform pain into pleasure in the physical, mental, and emotional realms – in every area of life. I know how to release old ideas easily and how to alchemize everything. I know who you really are and leading you to experience and to live in your real power feels like one of my greatest joys to teach.

Second, I have found ways beyond what science teaches, beyond what doctors are taught. I feel so amused at how so many doctors have not yet learned the simple yet powerful things I know. My experience has taught me things beyond what the culture, doctors, or even most scientists are taught or even imagine.

Speaking of gifts, I have found that my health issues have actually been a huge gift. I will share more about that later, but I feel trust that you will also find the incredible gifts that lay hidden under your pain and fatigue.

I feel so excited for you to step deeper into this book, for you to delve into these practices and do them with commitment and a sense of ease and fun. I feel so excited to hear how your body and your life transforms as you do these practices consistently.

Chapter 2:

What It Was like and What It's like Now

My fatigue and pain had cost me almost everything that I felt was important to me. I had been married to an extraordinary man, whom I still loved, but the longer we were married, the more tired, achy, stressed, and unhappy I got. I'd wake up feeling so achy. When we'd have an event or a date to go to, I would often be so sleepy I could not keep my head up. We would make a plan, but then I would feel so tired, I wouldn't be able to follow through. I'd say I was going to make dinner but then I would get so tired, I never made it, or I fell asleep as it was cooking and awoke to the scent of something burned.

All of this made me feel terrified. I felt so mad at myself. I would fall asleep and then I would get into an endless loop of beating myself up. I kept trying to find what was wrong with me.

I knew if I could solve this, I would be able to keep my life together. I knew if I solved this, life would feel worth living again.

My body ached all the time. I was constantly looking for something to ease the pain. I got massages twice a week when I could. I tried acupuncture, energy work, craniosacral massage, regular massage, deep tissue massage. I tried vitamins, changing my diet. I tried different types of exercise. I tried hypnosis. I tried immersing my body in immersion tanks. I went to all kinds of doctors. I tried herbs. I tried so many modalities I can't even remember most of them. I felt like my hormones were all over the place, and when I was on my cycle, I had cramps and even more fatigue.

When I ate certain foods, I would get nauseous. With some food, I had such an allergic reaction to it that I would have to go to the hospital to have my stomach pumped.

All my relationships were strained. My friends were absolutely fed up with my incessant fatigue. So many people told me they could not be friends with me anymore. That broke my heart. I remember falling asleep at a lunch that my dear friend took me to for my birthday and hers. I felt so ashamed. I wanted to make it up to her, but I didn't trust myself to be able to make a plan and she didn't trust me either.

I had not been able to work for a while. The last audition I went on before I found this solution felt awful. I actually fell asleep while the camera was on me. I felt like I wanted to crawl under the surface of the earth, I was so ashamed. I felt afraid to audition after that.

I felt hopeless. I felt like I would do anything to feel better.

My husband tried to be patient for years, but he couldn't handle it. Any time I started to get tired, unless it was at my normal bedtime, if he was with me, he'd get so angry. That terrified me, and I'd get more anxious and then more tired soon after.

I had wanted to be better with all my heart so he would love me again, but I couldn't find the cure and he didn't want to wait for me to get better anymore. We had separated and were in the process of divorce.

I was desperate to find a solution before he divorced me. I searched for anything I could find that might help. Some doctors told me they couldn't find what was wrong with me. One doc found that my adrenals were depleted – he said they were the most depleted adrenals he had seen in thirty years. He told me I may never recover. I was so devastated. I felt scared that I would never find another partner, never be able to work, and that I would end up on the street alone.

One night, everything changed. I felt so exhausted. My soon to be ex-husband was supposed to meet me for dinner – but he forgot.

Again.

I lay on the couch feeling so very sad. I couldn't stop crying. I felt so sick and tired. I didn't know what to do. I didn't have the energy to do anything. I couldn't even think to text him to remind him.

All I could think was that he didn't love me. He hated how I fell asleep so often. He hated how I was always late. I was late because I moved so slowly with all the pain and fatigue I had. I was late because I would have to pull my car over to take a nap on the way to meet him or take a nap before I left the house.

As I cried, I prayed. I asked for some guidance. I felt something pulling me as if from a string connected to my heart – to my bookshelf. My hand reached out and pulled out a book that I did not know I had. It was *The Law of Attraction*, by Jerry and Esther Hicks and Abraham.

I didn't remember buying it. I had never seen it before. But I remembered hearing someone talk about the book a few days before and I remembered her sharing how her life had turned around since reading it. I had made a mental note to buy it but had been too tired to do that. I felt so surprised to find this book on my shelf! I felt compelled to read it right then. Wiping my tears, I sat down and started to read…

The minute I read the first two chapters of the Law of Attraction, I felt a jolt of electric energy going up my body. I learned that my feelings let me know when I was in harmony with what I wanted or not. I learned that I could focus on a subject and by doing so sometimes I was creating what I wanted and sometimes I was pushing away what I wanted. I could tell if I was creating something I wanted because I would feel happy and I would be having fun. I could tell if I was creating what I did not want because I had negative emotions – I was afraid, nervous, judgmental, etc.

I realized I had been focused in a negative way on what I wanted. That's why I was getting the opposite of what I wanted!

I felt stunned. My whole life passed before my eyes and I realized that any time I was happy, playing with friends, having fun, or appreciating things, good things were coming to me and I had energy and felt pretty good – and any time I was complaining or scared or worried, I felt achy and tired and other bad things were happening. I saw it all so clearly. I felt amazed.

I had been complaining a lot. My life was at an all-time low. I was falling asleep everywhere, my friends and my ex-husband were mad at me for falling asleep so many times when we were at dinner or lunch or parties…

No one trusted me to be okay.

I felt depressed. I felt unsafe to drive. I was on the verge of falling asleep almost every time I drove.

I felt it clearly – my negative feelings were creating this terrible life. My negative feelings had destroyed my marriage and my health.

My feeling of trust in the knowing that the Law of Attraction was real was cemented at that moment.

I felt a glimmer of a spiritual awakening in that moment. I realized I needed to really understand the Law of Attraction. I realized I needed to change my focus… but I still had so much negative programming about every area of my life. I had so much past trauma that was still haunting me.

I would think of how I wanted my ex-husband back, but I would feel this incredible angst and tightness in my body. I felt so afraid and hurt by him.

I would think about my acting work and I would get belly cramps and be unable to breathe deeply.

The doctors had said I had depleted adrenals, a low thyroid, some food allergies, and narcolepsy. I felt tired and achy and my whole body hurt. My eyesight was failing me, my hair was getting thinner, my eyebrows had some empty spots in them. I was not a pretty picture!

I felt a strong desire within me to understand the Law of Attraction so I could get on track. I felt a speck of hope, but I also felt scared that I wouldn't be able to do it.

What if I couldn't get all this alignment that the book talked about? How would I learn it?

I joined a local Law of Attraction group, and that felt wonderful sometimes, but some people there complained more than they had fun.

I went to Abraham workshops, and Abraham complained about humans focusing on what they didn't want! I didn't understand. I felt so scared. How would I find my way?

What It's Like for Me Today

I feel like a totally new and vastly improved person. I feel amazed and beyond thankful for the transformation I have lived.

I just returned from an invitation-only expedition with one hundred world thought leaders to the high arctic to discuss the future. I felt honored to teach and lead morning meditations on the expedition boat. Many of these world thought leaders told me that my love and my meditations were one of the best things that happened on the trip. I felt boundless energy even though I was often the first person awake on the boat. The entire experience and the people I met felt so epic and beautiful.

Wonderful opportunities like this come to me all the time. I feel so blessed that I am constantly invited to meet extraordinary people and to experience wonderful things.

Today, and every day, I wake up feeling full of energy, full of love, full of pleasure. I have tapped into a chronic sensational, sensuous, sexy pleasure that I experience whenever I want, (and I want it all day every day! Giggle). It feels amazing to write this, or to work with clients, or drive, or sit down to eat, or cook, or fly on an airplane, or talk with someone, and to feel the incredible pleasure that dances through my body on a moment-to-moment basis. I feel I have found a pleasure trove!

In fact, as I write this, I feel incredible pleasure pulsing within me, just as I sit here and write. It's going up my spine, it feels like a gentle massage. This is one thing I will teach you that I have never seen anyone else talk about. It feels totally unique.

If I get any pain or injury, the pain is only there for a very short time – it feels like it's there for seconds or minutes or not at all. My body feels so drenched in pleasure that pain has no place to land anymore.

I feel beyond thankful for this tremendous gift.

I now have the energy to do whatever I want to. My friends who are half my age in the super fun dancing, singing yoga class I go to ask me how I got so energized. They often tell me that I have the energy of a happy three-year-old! (That feels so fun!) I can work long hours and feel fabulous. I can be out with friends or loved ones and feel vibrant, joyful energy easily as long as I want.

My doctor says I now have the physiology of a seventeen-year-old. I feel like a seventeen-year-old! My body looks about the same as it did when I was seventeen.

My energy throughout the day feels stable and steady. When I am asked if I am a morning person or a night person, I say yes, I am both. I am an afternoon person and I am energized any time of the day or night if I want to be. I just feel fabulous no matter what. And I love to get a good night's sleep, too. And if I do want a nap, it feels so luscious and perfect and energizing.

I feel so much love for exercise and I feel compelled to exercise. Exercising feels so fun! My body inspires me to move many times during the day in ways that keep me strong, supple, and energized. I feel thrilled to do my professional ski simulator, to do my whole-body vibration plate. I love to do handstands and to stretch with my yoga trapeze and on the floor. I feel amazing doing lots of exercises. If you saw one corner of my house, it totally looks like a super fun gym! My body is in better shape now than ever. My body looks the same as it did when I was a teenager (without the baby fat!). (And I have never done anything fake with my body – this is all from what I talk about in this book.)

I feel compelled to eat healthy, nourishing food. Without effort, food that did not serve me, like sugar, grains, caffeine, processed foods, GMO foods, and dairy, all fell away from me easily. I simply lost my desire for them. It feels so easy to eat fresh, organic, whole foods that this amazing planet provides and that really nourish my body and my brain.

My allergies all disappeared. I can now eat any food that I desire to eat, and my body stays happy.

My adrenal glands feel so calm and peaceful. My thyroid has become balanced and perfect. My skin has become clear, softer, smoother. My blood sugar has become totally stable. My menstrual cycle now brings me more pleasure, more comfort, and fabulous energy. My energy feels consistently good independent of my cycle now… My hormones feel totally balanced, naturally.

Twenty years ago, I used to wear glasses to read. Now I can read almost everything easily with no glasses. (I did not have any surgery on my eyes, nor medicine). This all happened naturally.

My hair has gotten thicker. My eyelashes have gotten longer and denser. My eyebrows filled in and are thick and healthy like when I was a kid.

I feel happy that I am always at the perfect weight. I never diet and my body just stays in a perfect balance. I wear the same size as when I was a teen (though my style has definitely changed!).

My suppleness and flexibility have increased. I can do stretches now that I have not done in years. I feel stronger than I have felt in years.

I feel no stress. Nothing feels challenging to me. I feel total peace and tranquility even when contrast comes. I feel tremendous trust in the perfection of all of life. If I get a little resistance, it is there for a few seconds, or even less, then I am back in the flow. And I love my resistance. I love all my emotions. I feel so much love for myself it feels epic. My mind feels tranquil, receptive, filled with the wisdom of the Universe. I feel invincible, unstoppable, I feel my eternal, infinite nature constantly and thoroughly. I feel blessed beyond measure. Life feels easy, simple, fun. I feel synchronicities happening all day every day.

People give me gifts wherever I go. People love to give me acts of service for free that thrill me. I feel so appreciative of who I am. I feel utterly confident and secure. I feel life loving me so very well.

I flow through life with utter relaxation and effortlessness. I have found the secret to driving easily in Los Angeles – it often seems like I am the only one on the road even at rush hour and I arrive so early now to most of my appointments.

My body feels healthier, younger, and more beautiful than ever. I often see my reflection in the mirror and simply gasp at the beauty I find in myself. I feel like I want to kiss myself all over, I love myself so much!

My relationships have all shifted to relationships of love and appreciation. I feel independent of the news, of what is happening in the world, yet I feel total love for the world.

I feel into the future and can feel the thrill of what is happening vibrationally already. My alignment feels solid. I trust myself completely.

I have found answers to every single situation I have encountered or that others have brought to me so far.

I feel so blessed that I often provide one-on-one coaching to coaches, psychologists, doctors, therapists, psychiatrists and other leaders and yet I watch them have one "aha" after another during our sessions. I feel amazed at all the wonderful things I have found that are unique and surprising to others.

Chapter 3:

The Path to Complete Well-being on Every Level

I feel so thrilled that these next pages will show you such a profound and fun and love-filled way to alchemize the fatigue and pain in your life into the vibrant energy and chronic pleasure you deserve.

I can break down my process into these ten steps:

1. **Applying the solution (Chapter 4)**

Many people are looking in all the wrong places for the solution. Here I give you the main solution and show you how you can start putting it into your body in a visceral way. Learn how to *feel* you are loved and supported in a visceral way, and how to access that love easily.

2. **Learn to apply the Law of Attraction in different areas for greater relief (Chapter 5)**

People often know the Law of Attraction intellectually, but they don't get it deeply into their body, nor do they apply that clarity in a deep way to all areas of their lives. I will show you how to do this.

3. **Transforming easily (Chapter 6)**

It's often tempting to stress over change or to try to force change, but real shifts happen effortlessly. When you tap into the effortlessness of transformation, you will feel excited to transform every area of your life.

4. Letting the Universe do the work (Chapter 7)

To really embrace the effortlessness of transformation, we find fun ways to allow the Universe to take care of things for you. As you get better at letting the Universe provide what you need, you release strain and tension and your body will thrive.

5. Changing cultural hypnotic suggestions (Chapter 8)

We are programmed from an early age by parents, teachers, our cultures, the news, TV and films, and so much more to believe in our limitations. Learning how to let go of the cultural conditioning will give you such a burst of energy and delight. You will feel a new power flow in.

6. Transforming every particle of life (Chapter 9)

Now it's time to find the often-hidden pockets that are adding to any pain or fatigue, and to release them. This chapter teaches you how to alchemize each area of your life so that it is beneficial to you and those around you.

7. Pleasure: the antidote to pain (Chapter 10)

As you learn to allow in the massive amounts of pleasure that are available to you, you actually rewire your brain in a way that makes pain almost impossible to experience. Pleasure is the antidote to pain. Pain simply becomes a one-sentence communication that tells you to move away from the fire, or sit with better posture, or walk to the left so as not to bump into that chair or take your wallet out of your back pocket when you drive so your hips are even. The more pleasure you experience, the more your body will communicate with you what it needs and block your pain and you will feel wonderful. And the more pleasure you feel, the more your energy will feel steady and reliable.

8. Nonphysical help (Chapter 11)

There is an entire stream of resources and support available to you that are easy to tap into. This chapter will also give you greater joy, which is a valuable part of good health.

9. Obstacles (Chapter 12)

Here we look at some of the areas of life that can be challenging, and I show you ways to transform them into solutions. If you try everything else I suggest, and you still have issues, this chapter should help.

10. What you learned (Chapter 13)

I will recap what you've learned and encourage you to take action in the best way possible. It will feel fun and easy and you will feel a new level of energy and pleasure.

My process actually feels fun and wonderful to do. And it's effective. If you follow these steps in the way I outline them, you will feel better and better. I have laid out every step that I used (except for those steps that are beyond the range of what can be explained in a book) to feel vibrant energy and chronic pleasure and I have detailed them here.

If you follow these steps, I feel totally certain you will feel little or no emotional or physical pain, more energized, more pleasure, and you will gain so many more blessings to each area of your life.

If you feel the desire to let go of emotional or physical pain and fatigue and to have more vibrant energy and more pleasure, then you are on the right path. Not everyone is drawn to a solution like this, but if this resonates with you, then definitely follow this fun, effective, pleasurable path! Stay committed to feeling vibrant energy and chronic pleasure. Know that it is totally possible. It is inevitable. It is certain. It is your birthright. Keep committed.

You were born to feel wonderful in your body.

Chapter 4:
Applying the Solution

O ur bodies are a reflection of our thoughts, emotions, and actions. In fact, our bodies respond to all of our thoughts, not just the thoughts about our bodies.

If you get upset at the news, that affects your precious body in a negative way. If you feel happy or are having fun, that's affecting your body in a positive way.

For me, I learned that I needed to be in alignment in every area of my life in order to let go of all my physical pain and to move into more and more pleasure (now I live in Chronic Pleasure) and to let go of all the fatigue I had to now have abundant energy.

I feel blessed to understand that every thought, every emotion, and every action is a prayer. If I am thinking thoughts that feel good, that is praying for what I do want. If I am thinking thoughts that are feeling bad, that is praying for what I don't want. I'll talk more about this later in the book, but for now, it'd feel awesome if you understand that everything you think, everything you feel, and everything you do is making you healthier or unhealthier in each moment. And your emotions help you discern this.

And that is a huge part of what this book is about. It's about transforming every area of your life so that you have pleasurable thoughts, pleasurable emotions, and good feeling actions that empower your body to feel its best, most happy, and most healthy.

I feel so fortunate – I have heard so many people say that they cannot be pure in positive thought, that they don't trust themselves to be able to be consistently positive, or that it's easy to forget about alignment, but for me, I have found that freedom of perpetual, consistent, easy alignment.

If I do get a negative thought, I recognize it so quickly that it simply falls away before it gets any negative momentum. And I always, ALWAYS remember that my connection with my Inner Being is the most important thing in my life.

In this chapter, I will give you some of my favorite practices for allowing yourself to first be aware of any negative thoughts, feelings, or actions, and then to learn to release them easily.

So, if you have any doubt that you can do this, I feel total understanding. I had that same doubt. But now I feel such faith. I have a freedom and such abundant health, and I feel excited for you to feel that too.

I encourage you to just relax, trust the process, and follow it as thoroughly as you can. You will be amazed at how much better you feel with each practice you do. And stay committed to yourself, stay committed to feeling good emotionally, so that, over time, your body will transform into feeling good too.

These practices and the clarity I am sharing are not meant to be done once and that's it. These are meant to be added into your life in a way that feels doable and easy, so that you can implement them daily or as often as you need for the rest of your life, until it all becomes automatic and effortless, like it has for me.

When you do them consistently, you actually encourage your brain to start helping you, and you also generate positive momentum so that the Universe can assist you in all you desire.

Your body or emotions did not get stressed, achy, and tired overnight. No, it's likely that anyone who has emotional or physical pain or fatigue has been practicing thoughts, feelings, and actions that haven't felt good for a while.

So apply these practices, these keys to your incredible good-feeling body with all the energy you need to do all you wish to do. And apply them with consistency.

To put this in a timeline, I practiced these things for months before I saw my first results… and then as I keep practicing them, my body has become healthier and happier. I feel younger and more agile, more capable than I have ever felt. I feel more pleasure every day. It feels incredible to be in my body now. I started this practice ten years ago as of this writing and it *keeps getting better* for me!!!

One last thing before we start: There is a huge paradox that trips many people up: *never do any of these practices in order to make anything happen. Do the practices because they feel so good to do. This is what I was talking about earlier in the book, when I said there is a way to do these practices that benefit your body and a way to do these practices that doesn't benefit you.*

If you are doing these practices (or anything) to heal your body, you are telling the Universe your body needs to heal, which then tells the Universe that you still have pain and fatigue. Also, you may do them out of obligation, which does not feel good, so it will backfire on your body.

However, if you do these practices (or anything) because they feel good to you, you will then feel good, which benefits your body.

Another aspect of this is that if you are doing something for a specific result, you may give up before you get the result. But if you are doing it because it feels good to do it, and you release the need for the result, your body will automatically get healthier and healthier. And you will be more likely to do it as a practice for the rest of your life too.

Heartfull Living

I feel that living in a state of unconditional love is what has healed my body.

The enlightened Persian poet, Rumi said, "Love is the Bridge between you and everything."

When you know how very easy it is to access the love that is here for you, you will feel so wonderful.

Having the heart be relaxed and open is the biggest key. That's why I teach all my clients how to be 'Heartfull' instead of 'Mindful.'

The wonderful scientists at HeartMath have found some amazing things about our extraordinary hearts. They found that:

"The heart sends more information from the nervous system to the brain than the other way around... The quality of the signals sent from the heart to the brain have tremendous effects on our brain function... [They] affect] our mental clarity, our emotions. The brain is largely interpreting the signals from the heart, to create how we feel... So if you can shift the rhythms of the heart, you can quickly improve brain function. You can quickly reduce stress, anxiety, [feeling] overwhelmed, but it takes a different doorway: the heart. When we get the systems in coherence, have the alignment between the heart and brain, that's when we access that deeper intuition that we have within, our inner guidance, so we have a new sense of clarity in a lot of decisions, that could seem complex otherwise."[1]

---

1   McCraty, Rollin, Science of the Heart, Exploring the Role of the Heart in Human Performance Volume 2. HeartMath® Institute. 2015. www.heartmath.org

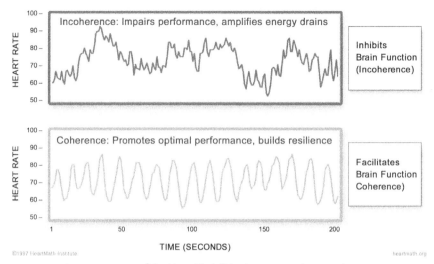

Image courtesy of the HeartMath® Institute – www.heartmath.org.

As you can see in the above picture, the feeling of coherence creates a much more steady, smooth and beautiful rhythm than incoherence.

To me, learning how to open my heart and to allow my heart to lead is one of the biggest gifts I have been given. And my soft open heart has been steadily retraining my brain to have improved thoughts so that now my brain is tranquil, quiet, and totally receptive to my inner genius.

HeartMath has also discovered that the heart receives information before the brain can hear it, see it, taste it, or touch it. Then the heart sends this signal to the brain and the brain interprets it and then communicates it to the body.

This first practice in this book gives you an experience of opening your heart and allowing yourself to be resourced, and then allowing your mind and body to relax and for all of you to be filled up with love. You receive love, which then makes it easy to give love. You are always receiving the love first, so loving is always easy. *When you are not trying to give first, you will have more energy right away.*

This is something I encourage you to practice many times a day so that you can really attune yourself to having a soft, open heart that is fully resourced.

NOTE: in this book, I will refer to that Divine aspect within each of us. I will use different phrases, like Inner Divinity, Inner Being, Source Energy, The Universe, Inner Brilliance, Inner Knowing, God... all of them mean the same thing. I mean that part of you that is in every particle of your body and in all of creation and beyond, and that knows all, loves all, and makes all whole. It's that part of you that knew how to take one sex cell from your dad and one from your mom and create a glorious, magnificent being like you with trillions of cells. It's the power that keeps the sun coming up daily. It's that energy that creates a tree from a tiny seed – and so much more.

If you have a particular way of naming that Divine Energy, then by all means, replace my names with your own. I honor all names of the Divine and all religions.

Practice 1. Heartfullness Meditation

1. Put your body in a relaxed and comfortable position. You can sit comfortably or lie down, whatever feels best. Bring your attention to your heart. If it helps you, gently rest your hand on your heart. Allow yourself to feel the beat of your heart. If you can't feel it, no worries – just put one hand on the pulse point on your wrist or your neck and feel the beat of your heart from there. Recognize that your heart is beating for you all the time. It beats when you are asleep, when you work, when you drive... your amazing heart is always taking care of you, working for you. Your amazing heart is always loving you.

2. Now imagine breathing softness, kindness, and warmth into your heart. Keep breathing it in and allowing your heart to be infused with that softness, that kindness, that warmth. Allow yourself to breathe in gentleness and relaxation. And let it infuse into your heart, like tea infuses into hot water.

3. As it infuses into your heart, feel your heart being soothed, softened.

4. As you feel this, your heart will be relaxing. Allow your heart to keep relaxing. And as it relaxes, it will open more and more. As your heart opens (I believe that your heart can open infinitely), it will be infused with that softness, that gentleness, that kindness that you have been breathing in.

5. And as you keep breathing in that gentleness, that kindness, that warmth, your heart will continue to open.

6. As your heart opens more and more, you may be able to *feel* the presence of your infinite, unconditionally loving Inner Being. This Inner Being is always there within you, it's always in your heart and in every particle of your brain and body, but it's easier to feel it when your heart is soft, relaxed, and open.

7. This Inner Divinity is within your heart, caressing your heart, nourishing your heart, softening your heart even more. You may feel the kindness, the love that your Inner Divinity has for you, as it nurtures your heart, soothes your heart.

8. As you feel this, recognize that you are loved no matter what you think, say, or do. You are loved so absolutely unconditionally by your Inner Being. Allow your heart to open and open and to be filled with the loving, kind, soothing presence of this Inner Being.

9. As your heart is being soothed and nurtured, it's automatically communicating with your precious brain that all is well. Your heart is letting your brain know that it too is filled with this infinite, unconditional, eternal love.

10. As your brain feels this, allow it to relax. Allow this Inner Divinity to soothe your brain, to caress it, to fill it with the true, infinite, eternal and unconditional love that is here for you.

11. As your brain allows this in, it will relax, it will let go, and it will open to the divine truth of your Inner Being. You may feel a new level of tranquility, peacefulness, calm.

12. And as your brain quiets, your brain is now communicating with your precious body that it, too, is filled with this pure love

of your Inner Divinity. You may feel this love nourishing your body, caressing your body, relaxing your body. You may feel your body tingling or feel the energy really loving each of your cells. You may feel your cells feeling lighter, happier, feeling like 'cell-ebrating' – giggle!

So now your heart is open, your mind is more relaxed, your body is relaxed, and you may be feeling pretty good.

This is the practice I would do over and over each day, sometimes eight or thirteen or more times each day, so that I would practice feeling my heart being open and soft. I would do this when I felt good or when I felt bad – it took a bit longer for me to feel my heart open and my mind get tranquil when I felt bad, but either time, it would give me a greater awareness of the state of my heart.

Now, I keep my attention on my heart throughout the day and I feel it filled up consistently with an abundance of love. This has made my ability to love myself and others unconditionally much easier. And it makes me more aware when I feel my heart starting to close. If I feel that, I immediately begin this soft breathing into my heart, and I do the above steps until I am back in alignment. Having practiced this for years, it now happens almost unconsciously so that I feel in steady, consistent flow and filled with love all the time.

I encourage you to practice this many times each day. If you don't feel significantly better after trying this the first time or two, that's okay, don't give up. This is a practice that gets better with each time you do it. It will become a source of great soothing for you if you practice this enough. And you too, will find a greater awareness of your precious heart and its ability to influence your brain into a state of tranquil loving calm.

How does this help your body? When your heart is wide open, when you feel loved, when your mind is open, relaxed, and receptive and your body feels easy, you are creating a perfect fertile ground for your body to do its genius work to bring about the health and well-being you desire– with you out of the way.

Each time you allow yourself to fill up entirely with the infinite, unconditional, eternal love that your Inner Divinity has for every particle of you, you are also creating new patterns in your brain that are patterns of ease, of well-being, of love. And as you feel this more and more consistently, you can influence your genetic expression so that you are more likely to be expressing the genes of well-being and health. Consistency is the practice. It's really about doing this so consistently that your body has a chance to get back into its own brilliant rhythms and bring you the relief from pain and the energy you crave.

Stress is one of the leading causes of all diseases, so the more you practice this, the more you will be training your heart, body, and brain to let go of stress and to be more coherent and aligned, which will cause your pain to be released and your energy to soar.

A Beautiful Example of the Power of HEARTFULLNESS:

My client, Gonzalo, is a therapist in Spain. He was taught that he had to feel negative emotions to release them. I began to take him through this Heartfull Meditation practice and he stopped me, saying that his mind was very critical and it wouldn't be quiet. I coached him for a few minutes, and I led him through this practice again. This time he went deep. He totally relaxed into the love from his heart. He told me he felt connected to himself for the first time and his mind had been quiet and receptive.

This is what he wrote me after our work together:

"A long time ago a friend told me, 'There is a woman who lives like a goddess on earth.'

Nothing was more interesting to me than to investigate who she is (you), and I did, on Facebook and YouTube.

I'm so sensitive to energies, to the pureness, and I felt immediately that you were a living example of the energy I wanted to be and to incarnate. Your example told me that my ideal energy state was possible.

The next step was to find out how you became that way. I asked you a few times, I saw your videos, I did your meditations, and finally, I was ready for a session with you.

The session was one of the most powerful tipping points in my life. It made me find one of the missing pieces and fit the puzzle, and to start a new way in my life, with your meditation, expanding, even more, my heart energy.

The day of our session I experienced for the first time, the experience of unconditional love. And I learned, I think by osmosis or your [Karen's] example, that it was possible. I keep doing the meditation you made for me every day. Now it's a hobby, or an exciting activity for me. Now I love to meditate.

Now I live in an amazing synchronicity, I'm an impassioned human being. I bring laughter energy to earth. And I remember my decision before I was born to explore the extreme of darkness and laugh in the darkness. And of course, in the light. I am doing so.

Things are getting better and better. Knowing that no matter what happens, it only matters what I do with what happens gives me the permission to live in the moment without worrying.

Every time that a contrast arises, automatically my heart opens, and I am laughing with my situation and my energy embraces that negativity and easily transforms the energy to what I prefer – and I prefer joy. You

*do something similar, but you do it soooo much faster
than me and in a Karen style and way.*

*The issue that inspired me to reach out to you was to
live with the heart open. Thank You Very Muchísimo,"
Gonzalo Vidal Páez"*

I love my work!

Relevant: How to Know What to Focus Upon

My amazing, wonderful love-filled, funny, fun mom is Greek, so
I grew up learning the etymology of words since I was a little girl. I
always feel excited looking up the etymology of words, which is why
one day, when I was thinking about the word "relevant," I got inspired
to look up the etymology.

The word "relevant" has one etymology that comes from the Latin,
"relevare," which originally meant to raise or lift up, to lessen or to
lighten, to relieve.

The moment I realized that the things that lifted me up and lightened
me, the things that relieved me, were relevant, I felt a massive shift.

I saw all the things I had been taught, the things I heard on the
news, the things I heard from doctors, from school, from friends… and
I could feel that so many of them did not lift me up and lighten me.

In that moment, I felt my Inner Being within me saying that the
reason thoughts that are relevant feel like I am being lifted up and
lightened, the reason they feel like relief, is because that is an indication of my greater alignment with all that I want. It's is a sign that I
am on track.

I felt the clear knowing that unless a thought lifted me up and lightened me, unless a thought gave me relief, it *could not be true*, because
only those thoughts that lift me up and lighten me are true. Thoughts
that lift me up and lighten me are true because my Inner Being sees the

bigger picture and knows the *real truth*. And my Inner Being gives me that good feeling to let me know I am on track.

In that moment, I was able to release a lifetime of irrelevant thoughts and beliefs. They just fell away effortlessly. And when I encounter anyone telling me something that does not lift me up or lighten me, now I know I can relax, open my heart, and just let myself open to a deeper truth, a more relevant knowing that my Inner Being will give me.

Practice 2. Relevant: Focusing on What Lifts You up and Lightens You

It'd feel good if you start examining the beliefs or thoughts you have to see if they lift you up and lighten you or not. Look especially at the thoughts and beliefs you got from doctors, teachers, the news, family, friends, and especially the thoughts you tell yourself about yourself… basically look at what you believe from *every area*!

Look to see how it feels when you focus on each thought or belief. If it feels good, if you feel lighter and happier when you think it, it's a keeper for now. If it feels bad, or if it limits you in some way, it cannot be the Divine Truth and so you can realize it's a lie, it's a false belief, and you can simply let it go. And as you get more and more aligned, some of the beliefs that did lift you up and lighten you before will soon become irrelevant and you will find new, more high-flying beliefs.

For example, I used to feel lifted up and lightened by the thought that everything is working out for me. Now that feels like a low vibration for me and now I feel lifted up and lightened by the thought that I am receiving everything I want in every moment.

Get out a piece of paper or open your notes on your phone or computer and write down the beliefs that you feel lift you up and lighten you now.

If they really make you feel better, then you can read this list of relevant, light, raised up thoughts over and over. The more you read them, the better you will feel. And you can add to them as you find new, happier thoughts and this will become a list of wonderful-feeling ideas that you can refer to any time you want to feel better.

When you feel a thought that does not lift you up and lighten you, you can know it's not the Divine Truth and this is when you can bring in the first practice, the Heartfullness Meditation, by starting to breathe softness into your heart and connecting with your Inner Divinity, and allowing your heart to receive that energy and to flow it out to your mind and body. As you do that, greater clarity is likely to flow in.

For me, having kept my heart soft and open for years, if anything negative comes to me, I feel an immediate knowing of a deeper Divine Truth that really thrills me.

And the negative thought or belief vanishes.

If you practice this enough, you will get that same inner knowing of Divine Truth that is right for you, and you can then add that new knowing to the list of relevant thoughts.

Self-Love

Loving yourself is one of the keys to feeling better physically. When you really love yourself, you are kind, gentle, and soothing with yourself. You will find that you become inspired toward the foods, exercises, people, experiences, and actions that are right for you. You will find that you are more and more in the right place at the right time in the right way. And your body will feel greater and greater relief from pain, and more and more energy.

I play two fun games with my body and myself that increase my self-love.

The first game I use is a modified version of the Alphabet Game, which I learned from Esther and Jerry Hicks and Abraham. (Thank you!)

I call it my *ABC Self-Love Game*.

My version starts with the letter A, and I look for A words that lift me up and lighten me and I add in the beginning statement, 'I feel' or 'I have' or 'I am'… For example, I say, "I feel Awesome, I am Answers, I feel Adventurous, I feel Agile, I feel Ageless, I have abundance…" and I go on and on and on until I cannot think of any more A words that lift me up and lighten me. I only use words that lift me up and lighten me.

Then I go with B: "I am Beautiful, I feel Blissful, I feel Bountiful. I feel Brilliant. I feel Blessed. I have blessings." And I go on and on and on until I cannot think of any more B words that lift me up and lighten me.

And I keep going through the alphabet as long as I can to the end. It can take a couple of hours if you really play with this, but those hours are intoxicatingly fun.

I would do this while I drove, and I would find myself getting around Los Angeles faster and more easily.

Later in the book, I will talk about moving in the flow in any city.

The more I played, the better my body felt. I got tremendous energy and I began to experience more and more pleasure as I played. It felt like I got so giddy playing this. I feel so high naturally from this game!

I have also played this game with friends. We would each say the 'I am or I feel or I have…' phrase about ourselves and we'd feel giddy and intoxicated by the time we got to the letter C. Whoever wants to just jumps in to share what they feel they are or have or do and we just go around the circle saying things in random order. It feels so fun.

A Fun Real-Life Example

One friend that I played this ABC Self-Love Game was an Internal Medicine doctor at USC Hospital.

George felt so high after playing this game with me that he took it to his work, where he was seeing patients and teaching residents how to be doctors.

First, he started playing it with his residents and they were more attentive, relaxed, and positive with the patients. George told me they had more confidence in doing supervised procedures (which I am sure the patients appreciated, too!).

And George told me how he had one patient who was under his care and he had just gotten some bad news about his health. George told his patient about this game. He told him that he knew that his patient's test results had been bad, but he encouraged his patient to just forget about that for that time and just play this ABC Self-Love Game until George came back from his rounds.

George went on his rounds. When he returned about ninety minutes later, that patient who had been playing the ABC Self-Love Game had a big smile on his face and looked more relaxed. The patient said he felt so much better.

The better one feels emotionally, the better the body feels physically.

After hearing George's enthusiastic reports, I felt committed to playing that ABC Self-Love Game with myself and others forever.

Practice 3. ABC Self-Love Game

This ABC Self-Love Game is only good to play when you are already feeling good.

If you don't feel good, go back to Practices 1 and 2 (the Heartfullness Meditation and the Relevant Practice) and do those. When you feel better and your heart is open, when your mind is more receptive and you feel loved, that's a better time to play.

You can write out the 'I am, I feel, I have' phrases for each letter. You can also play this when you drive or do anything where you can focus on something else. I often do it as I am falling asleep. And it may feel fun to do when you are with a group of friends or family. I often do it with my mom while we go for a walk. When we get to the Bs she always says, "I feel Bodacious." That feels hilarious coming from my sweet, gentle mom!

It felt so bonding when four of us who were new friends were at lunch and we decided to play the game. We were four people from 4 different countries with 4 different languages. Everyone said their phrases in English and in their languages. We were laughing so hard.

I felt intoxicated by the joy and they all did too. Everyone said it was the most connected, giddy meal they had ever had. None of us wanted to leave.

It feels like we can't stop laughing at all the hilarious things we come up with. It feels so playful and light and soothing to play this game as long as you are doing it just because it feels enjoyable, not to make anything happen, but because it feels so good emotionally. That's the attitude for each of these practices.

The second game I play is called *Flirting with my Body*.

I often do this when I am just waking up and am in the sleepy dreamy state, or when I am in the shower.

If I am in bed, I relax myself deeply and then I start with my feet (though you can start anywhere) and I go up my body and tell each part of my amazing body how much I love it.

I tell my body it is brilliant. I tell it I am so proud of it. I tell each part of my body that it is valuable and precious and that I cherish it. I tell my body it is beautiful. I tell my body I feel admiration for it.

I flirt with my body until I am at the point where I want to kiss myself all over. (This feels like pure delight!)

After I have done this, I have often caught a glimpse of myself in the mirror and I gasp at my radiance. It's a sure radiance booster!

My body and yours *love* to be celebrated, appreciated, approved of, and admired.

Practice 4. Have Fun Flirting with Your Body!

You can do this practice any time you are feeling good. If you are not feeling good, go back to the first and second practice (the Heart-fullness and Relevant practices) and do those. Or get a bite to eat of healthy, nourishing food, or pet your cat, or take a nap, or do anything that makes you feel better emotionally.

When you feel lifted up and lightened, if you can, relax yourself deeply, then start going through each part of your body.

Praise it.

Admire it.

Celebrate it.

Be proud of it as it is now and as it is becoming.

Whisper sweet somethings into the ears of your cells.

Know that your body is listening to your thoughts *all the time*, so the more consistently you do this, the more your body will feel its own brilliance and it will feel your Inner Divinity doing things that will improve the way your body feels in every way.

Both of the practices in this section are meant to be done in a consistent way, so keep playing.

You may find yourself getting so romantic with your body as you keep flirting that you will fall so deeply in love with yourself, and you will forever be kind, gentle, and loving to your amazing body and self.

I wrote this poem for you:

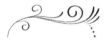

Have you looked at yourself lately?
Oh my!
Your beauty feels so magnificent,
I feel astounded and just want to congratulate you for
your Mastery!
You shine so brightly, that I feel in awe of your fortunes.
Eagles swoon when they catch sight of you!
Dolphins leap with joy when you are anywhere near!
Flowers exude their loving fragrance
so you can be sure
you are welcome when you pass them by.
If you cannot see this unspeakable glory in yourself,
try looking at yourself from My Eyes.
Your heart will break open
and you will bow at your own magnificence!

And you will forever after
be
gentle,
kind,
soothing
and
loving
to yourself!
By Karen Lorre

Chapter 5:

Learn to Allow Yourself to Feel Loved Easily

Because our body is a reflection of our thoughts, including our thoughts about others and the world, it is important to shift any areas that may not be lifting you up and lightening you.

As I became aware of all the qualities of Love, I started to put each quality of Love into practice. My life became more and more magical and I felt my body loving this practice and showing me that it loved it by being more energized and feeling more pleasure.

Feeling Approved of and Validated

Many people feel the need to be approved of and validated, but this creates an endless negative loop, because most humans cannot approve of and validate someone unconditionally and certainly not 24/7. We all need to sleep!

And when we look for approval or validation from outside of ourselves, we find that it never really goes deep enough.

I had such a deep need to be approved of that I could not function well without external validation. This really strained my health and made me feel so fatigued. It made it hard for me to make decisions. I felt estranged from my intuition. And my relationships did not fare well!

Then one day, as I was using my credit card to pay for my groceries. I saw the credit card machine say the words, 'Approved.'

In that moment, I felt my Inner Being telling me that I was approved of unconditionally.

I felt my whole body shake with tears of relief as I allowed that in.

I felt my Inner Being telling me that the Entire Universe approves of me. I started to feel this energy of approval, of being validated flowing into every particle of my body while I was still at the check stand.

I left the store and went into my car and cried with a deep sense of letting go and allowing in this epic, infinite, eternal approval and validation, this validation and approval that is unconditional, and that is actually flowing into us 24/7.

From that moment on, my need to receive approval and validation from others vanished. I now feel that I am completely approved of – unconditionally. I feel completely validated no matter what I am doing, feeling, or thinking.

Once I had this clarity, I practiced feeling it everywhere.

My biggest desire has been to love as my Inner Being loves. So, when I felt this unconditional approval, I also wanted to feel it for myself and for the world.

The first time I decided to try to approve of everything outside of me, I was driving on Pacific Coast Highway in Malibu, California. I saw the beautiful ocean and I approved of it, I saw the trees and the mountains, and I approved of them. I saw all the other drivers driving and I approved of them. I saw I was slouching as I drove, and I approved of myself and sat up straighter.

Then, I was still driving, and a truck moved in front of me. This truck had a fake scrotum hanging under the bumper. I felt an immediate lack of approval, then I breathed softness into my heart, I relaxed my mind and body. A moment later, I felt so much laughter shaking my belly, and I felt my ability to approve open up.

I felt thankful for that truck owner for his inspiration that opened up my ability to approve more than I had previously thought was possible.

And I keep practicing approval of *everything*.

When I was tired and needed a nap, I would feel this approval, I would hear my Inner Being tell me in a very soothing, approving way that I was right on track, that it was perfect I was taking a nap, that it was the best thing I could do, that when I woke up, I would feel better and I could then transmute whatever it was that had been bothering me that made me tired (more about that later) and I would approve of myself, basically copying my Inner Being's words to myself.

If I had any pain, I would approve of it. I would hear my Inner Being tell me that I could feel thankful that this pain was communicating what it needed with me. I would hear from my Inner Being that I could tell this pain that I loved it as it was, that it never needed to change, I would accept it as it was. I practiced approving of any pain in the same way.

When I felt or said or did something out of alignment, I approved of myself. I would hear my Inner Being saying that all of my emotions and actions are valuable, they teach me if I am in alignment or not, and that when I feel any emotions, I can just love them all and approve of them as they are. I heard my Inner Being tell me that approval causes negative emotions to soften and to disappear.

When I saw someone doing something I did not want, I relaxed and practiced approving of them. Another time I saw a man who was sleeping on the grass on the side of the road. I asked my Inner Being how my Inner Being felt about him. In that moment, I felt so much love, my heart felt like it was overflowing with this luscious warmth and softness. I saw the goodness, the value, the worthiness of this beautiful man. Now I feel that about *everyone*.

This affected my body and my whole being in an amazing way. My naps got fewer and farther apart, I started to feel more and more energy. My body was letting go of pain in a rapid way. I felt healthier overall. And my heart felt more and more like it was shining brighter and brighter with each moment of approval.

If you cannot hear your Inner Being guiding you on how to approve of yourself just yet, that's okay, it is totally understandable. I have been meditating twenty-eight years (as of this writing) nearly every day, which really helps me to attune to the more subtle communications from the Divine. My ability to discern the subtle voice of my Inner Being feels pretty refined and it keeps getting better.

The more open your heart and the quieter your mind the more you will hear or feel or see your Inner Being. You are welcome to use the words I heard or to find other soothing things to say to yourself. The more you practice this, the easier it will be to feel this wonderful feeling of knowing you are right on track, that you are perfect as you are now, and you are perfect as you move into greater and greater alignment.

Practice 5. Practicing Feeling Approved of and Validated

Do Practice 1, Heartfullness Meditation, and when you feel your whole body and mind are relaxed, tune into your heart and ask your Inner Being to let you feel how approved of you are.

Recognize that you are approved of by your Inner Being and by the Entire Universe unconditionally. Recognize that the Entire Universe is always validating you.

Allow the reassuring, validating energy of being approved of to drench your amazing heart, to permeate your brilliant mind, to saturate your precious body.

Feel the gentle, validating, soothing energy of approval flowing into you from every direction.

As you practice feeling this over and over, gently start to apply it to every part of yourself.

Practice telling your beautiful body that you approve of it. Practice telling your mind that you approve of it.

Practice approving of yourself unconditionally.

Practice approving of your body unconditionally.

Approve of yourself when you are in or out of alignment.

Approve of your body when it's tired or feeling pain.

Approve of your negative emotions.

Once you have practiced feeling approved of and validated, then you can practice feeling and flowing approval to everyone in your path.

This is not a serious thing. It can be played like a game of 'Can I approve of this? Can I approve of that?'

Allow this game to feel playful, light, and wonderful as you keep opening your heart to a bigger and bigger capacity to approve, validate, and love. Practice approving of yourself and the people in your life unconditionally, no matter what they do.

The more you practice this feeling, the better your body will feel! And your relationships will thrive, too!

Approval in Action with My Wonderful Client, Teri

My amazing client Teri did coaching and meditation sessions with me. During one session, I coached her about approving unconditionally and suggested she approve of everything she could. This is what she wrote me:

"Karen!! I am so loving this approving of every-thing I got from the guided meditation you made me!! I'm making a game out of it and it is so freeing!! Even for silly things like someone cutting me off in traffic, I'm approving of it!! It feels so free!! I now get what it means to mind my own business. It really doesn't matter at all what other people are thinking, just what I am thinking!!! I love it!! This morning I had sniffles and approved of it. In the past, I used to resist it and

wonder what I was doing wrong to create it and just think about it a lot. Since I approved of it, it's passing right through me quickly and almost gone!

Since our coaching session, things are really flowing. The right people and the right timing, just flowing. I never realized how easy this could be! And the best part is it keeps getting better and I know all it can do is get better and better!! Thank you again so much!!!"

Teri Thomas (NY)

Feeling Understood

I used to lament how no one understood me. I was constantly telling people, "You never understand me!" I felt hopeless. I could never seem to find a way for people to really get who I was, for people to trust my good intentions.

Then one day I felt totally surprised and delighted as I realized that the Entire Universe understood me perfectly. The Universe understood me so well that it was bringing me people who did not understand me! My belief that no one understood me caused the Universe to bring me people who did not understand me! This was the Law of Attraction working with what I believed! I felt amazed. I felt so much laughter bubbling up as I grew lighter with this awareness. The laughter came because I felt so happy I had created it and I knew I could shift this easily.

I began to practice saying to myself that everyone understands me. And little by little, as I practiced this and repeated it silently over and over, I started to believe it. As I believed it, more and more people understood me completely. And the more I practiced believing that people understood me, the more connected to others and to myself I felt, the more I felt seen for who I truly am. Now many people really see who I am right away. And of course, the more I did this, the more my body started to feel better and better. It felt so easy.

And an added benefit was that as I felt understood, my ability to understand others increased which made all my relationships feel better too. YAY!

Practice 6. Practice Feeling Understood

Allow yourself to recognize that the Entire Universe understands you. You may see patterns of thought you have had and how the Universe has been bringing you just what you have been focused upon. You are a powerful creator!

Do Practice 1, Heartfullness Meditation, and when you feel your mind and whole body are relaxed, tune into your heart and ask your Inner Being to let you feel how understood you really are. Allow the soft beautiful energy of being understood to drench your amazing heart, to permeate your brilliant mind, to saturate your precious body.

As you practice feeling this over and over, gently start to apply it to every part of yourself. Practice telling your beautiful body that you understand it, practice telling your mind that you understand it.

Feel the knowing that you are getting whatever it is you predominantly think about, whether you want it or not. You can change your thoughts by practicing new thoughts. As you practice a new thought, you start to change yourself and your world.

Start practicing saying silently that this person understands you and that person understands you. Start practicing saying that *you* understand you.

As you practice this, you will feel yourself relaxing more and more. And relaxation is key for releasing pain and having more energy.

Practice saying how you understand others. Practice feeling how you understand life, how you understand how to do or be or have anything you want. You get what you focus upon so let yourself practice fun-feeling new ideas. Practice feeling and flowing understanding to everyone in your path.

A note about practice: to me, practice means repetition, but repetition in a fun, playful way. Simply repeating something in a way that feels good or feels fun is how I practice everything that feels important to me, or I get myself super relaxed and practice it in that sensual way. So, practice thinking thoughts that feel good and keep repeating the same good feeling thoughts.

Here's a playful example of how the Universe understood me.

One day, I felt the knowing that I was really a Goddess. I felt so excited about that clarity. I felt inspired to practice telling myself, "I am a Goddess." I said it over and over for about three days. On the third day I was inspired to take a walk – wearing a dress and high-heeled boots. That's not my normal walking in the neighborhood style, but I listened to my inspiration.

I found myself in front of a restaurant. I had already eaten a late lunch and it was only about 5 p.m. and I was not feeling hungry. But I felt almost as if I was being energetically pushed into the restaurant. Inside, the restaurant was pretty full. It only had community seating and there were only two available seats. The host was offering me either of the seats, but I felt my whole body pushed into the first seat.

I was sitting at a table with about eleven other people.

The woman next to me started to talk with me. Her name is Lisa Levart. She was there with her husband, Myles, and a dear friend of theirs, Liz Benjamin, but Myles and Liz were talking to each other, so she had turned to connect with me. As we talked, I fell in love with her immediately. I was beaming love and joy at her. We connected on so many wonderful levels.

After we had spoken for a bit, Lisa said, "You are exuding such love, such joy… I do Goddess Portraits. Would you like to be one of my Goddesses?"

Inside my body, I could feel my heart leaping. "Yes!"

Two days later Lisa photographed me as the Goddess Aphrodite in Malibu. Lisa posted it in the *Huffington Post*. You can view the article here: http://bit.ly/2JmEwd7

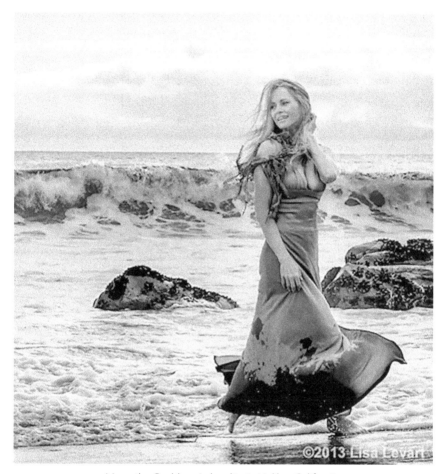

Me as the Goddess Aphrodite in Malibu, California.
Credit © 2013 by Lisa Levart / www.goddessonearth.com/goddesses

Then a friend of mine that I did not know worked at the Huffington Post, Lance Khazie, emailed me saying he had seen the article and asked if we'd like to do a Huff Post Live event about Goddesses.

I felt excited! "Yes!"

So Lisa Levart, Agapi Stasinopoulos, Gloria Feldt, and I were interviewed about being Goddesses on Huff Post Live.

Here's the link if you want to watch it: http://www.goddessonearth. com/huff-post-live-interview

Then the Master Artist to the Dalai Lama, Romio Shrestha, came over (I was given a tibetan *thangka* of his, White Tara, the Goddess of Compassion, and that's how we met). I feel so thankful that the person who gave it to me knew I was a Goddess of Compassion.

Romio said he was doing a documentary called *1000 Goddesses* and he asked if I'd be one of his Goddesses. I have filmed my part for this documentary, my part of the documentary is now on YouTube. So again, I was a Goddess for his documentary.

Then Lisa Levart returned to Los Angeles and we decided to do another Goddess portrait. I became the Goddess Lila. (Lila is not really a Hindu Goddess – the word "Lila" means playfulness in Sanskrit – so I decided to make that playful energy into the form of a Goddess. I wanted to be Lila.)

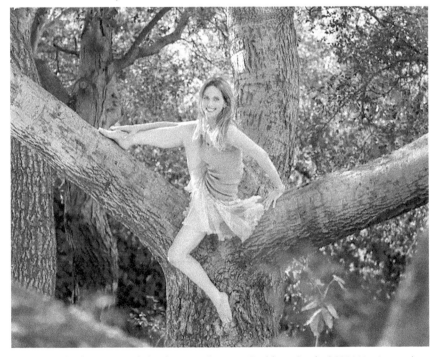

Me as Lila, the energy of play that I made into a Goddess. Credit ©2016 Lisa Levart / https://www.huffingtonpost.com/lisa-levart/i-just-want-to-have-fun_b_8908214.html

I just returned from Paris, and so many people I met there said, "*Tu es une déesse*," which translates to, "You are a Goddess." That felt so beautiful and I heard it from the people at the farmers market and the stores on the street where I was staying and from the new friends I met.

The Universe really does understand me. When I believed that no one understood me, no one understood me. When I believed that I am a Goddess, the Universe showed me that I am a Goddess. Giggle.

The Universe understands anything you say about yourself, or about another or about the world, and it is bringing it to you. Look for places in your life where you have a practiced belief and see how the Universe is bringing you just that. If you like what you are getting, keep practicing it, but if not, start practicing thoughts that really lift you up and lighten you. Practice saying, thinking, and feeling only happy thoughts about the things that you want.

One further application of this trick: I used to be very computer illiterate. I would have to go to the Apple Genius Bar so often. My computer was always having challenges. Then I heard my negative thoughts about my computer abilities, and I got excited to change them. I practiced believing that I understood my computer and I am a tech genius. I don't have an interest in writing code, but my ability to find solutions on my own for my computer got better and better and better. My computer genius friend, Marc, actually called me a Tech Ninja because I find solutions so fast now!

Feeling Accepted

One day, as I was focusing on what love feels like, I felt the feeling of "Acceptance" pouring into me. I felt this kind, loving, gentle acceptance of me flow into my body. It felt so sweet, I felt my heart expand. As it flowed, I felt my shoulders drop and my breathing deepen. I felt sweet tears of appreciation for this wonderful feeling of being accepted unconditionally. I felt my whole body begin to relax deeper.

As I continued to practice feeling accepted in a sweet, fun way, I also started to practice accepting myself, accepting my resistance, accepting the world as it is, and accepting others.

All the efforts I had been using to control or to fix or to change things fell away.

I could feel that with this depth of being accepted and then turning this feeling out toward my world around me, I was dropping tons of resistance.

I accepted myself exactly as I am. I accepted my body exactly as it is. I accepted my life exactly as it is. I accepted the people in my life exactly as they are.

As I accepted everything, I could see the beauty in me, in everyone. I could feel the perfection, the magnificence in me and everyone. I felt a deep peacefulness and relaxation slowly seep its way into my whole being as I practiced feeling this wonderful feeling. It felt like my bones were being filled with such a strong, beautiful energy of acceptance. I felt stronger and softer at the same time.

I had the concern that if I accepted everything maybe nothing would change, but then I felt the knowing that if I accept everything, I am no longer pushing against anything, and now I am allowing myself and my body and my life and those in my life to be free to be who they truly are.

All of my relationships improved. And my health continued to thrive in a much more relaxed, effortless way. My body filled with more pleasure. My energy kept increasing.

Now it feels so easy to accept what is, and yet also focus on what I want (more about that a bit further into the book).

Practice 7. Feeling Accepted

Do Practice 1, Heartfullness Meditation. When you feel your whole mind and body are relaxed, tune into your heart and ask your Inner Being to let you feel how accepted you are. Allow the kind, gentle, soothing energy of acceptance to flow into your extraordinary heart, to saturate your receptive mind, to envelop and drench your incredible body.

As you practice feeling this over and over, gently start to apply it to every part of yourself.

Practice telling your beautiful body that you accept it as it is. Practice telling your mind that you accept it as it is.

Feel how you are accepted when you have resistance. Feel how you are accepted when you do or feel or think something out of alignment.

There is no time that you are not accepted. You are accepted by the Entire Universe all the time. You belong to this wonderful Universe and the Universe belongs to you. You are welcomed, allowed to be as you are, totally accepted by this loving Universe no matter what you do. It is flowing into you unconditionally.

When you feel like you are fully accepted, that you are drenched in this amazing feeling of being accepted, and you can feel the unconditionality of it, then start allowing that acceptance to flow out to the others in your world and to the entire world. Practice feeling and flowing acceptance to everyone in your path. Accept the things you hear about in the news. Accept the things that formerly gave you resistance. Accept your resistance. Accept the resistance of others…

As you are flowing the acceptance you receive, you will be in greater peace, greater tranquility. You will feel a new freedom, a new power flowing in as you practice allowing in and flowing this rich, beautiful feeling of acceptance. Your body will enjoy a deeper relaxation and therefore deeper health and well-being.

Later on, we'll talk about envisioning what you want. When you accept everything and envision what you want with the intention of feeling good in this moment, you become unstoppable.

Feeling the Universe Proud of You

Have you felt the need to accomplish something spectacular before you can feel proud of yourself or before you feel worthy of others feeling proud of you? Did you grow up feeling you were not good enough? That you don't measure up to some external parent or religion or partner or teacher's vision of you? Have you tried to work very hard to make someone outside of you proud of you? Or do you have the belief that we should be humble and that feeling proud of ourselves is arrogant?

If so, you are in luck today!

All of this effort and negative emotion takes a huge toll on the body. But there is a way to bypass all that negative programming easily. Read on, my dear, beloved!

An Example from One of My First Clients

As I was coaching one of my very first clients for the first time, I tuned to his Inner Being and I immediately felt how the Universe and his Inner Being were so proud of him. I had never felt that before and I felt amazed. It felt unmistakable that the whole Universe was so proud of him. There was no denying it. I put that into his meditation recording.

This is what he wrote to me after our session:

"Karen Lorre's Guided Meditations are a gift from a higher dimension. Words simply don't do justice to the experience. It's as though she's able to make a comfortable yet direct connection to a deep part within you that then guides the meditation.

As she gently reflects back the words you need to hear, you first fall into a deep relaxation. As the meditation deepens, what follows can only be described as a slow, steady, rich crescendo toward your own greatness. What's still amazing is that, without really knowing me at all, she was able to use words and phrases that have very specific and important meaning to me. When we were done, I felt as though I had taken a jour-

ney deep within myself and then returned as a more self-aware and self-empowered person. Every time I listen, I experience a deeper knowing and allowing. I'm eagerly anticipating my next Guided Meditation experience with Karen."

Kevin Young (Michigan)

After I had done that session with Kevin, I felt the Universe being proud of me too, all the time. I could feel my non-physical dad, telling me he was so proud of me. It felt amazing. I felt tears of appreciation flowing as I let this wonderful feeling of him and the Entire Universe feeling proud of me sink in. I felt so rich as it flowed in. It felt like the Universe being proud of me was filling in all these tiny empty pockets in my body with a warm, powerful, supportive energy that I had unconsciously been craving. I felt the Universe being proud of what I had accomplished even when to me, I felt I had accomplished very little.

Then I heard the Universe tell me that it was proud of me, of you, of everyone, unconditionally. I heard the Universe tell me that this feeling of it being proud of us is not ego-based, it is simply the recognition of our incredible magnificence. I heard that real humility is recognizing the absolute magnificent splendor of who you are and of who everyone else is. I felt so amazed.

Once I felt that feeling of the Universe being proud of me steadily, I started to take what I received and flow it out to the world.

I practiced feeling proud of people in the news, of things I did not like, of violence in the world.

It's not that I wanted more of that, but I wanted my heart to keep opening wider and wider so I could be more and more pure in my love. That's why I wanted to feel proud of those things I did not want. I did not stay thinking of them very long, I simply let that feeling of being proud of them flow to them and then I moved on.

Since this time, my beautiful non-physical dad keeps coming, making me feel how very proud of me he is. I always feel my heart saturated with his love when I feel that. I am feeling that now. Tears are flowing as I write this.

Practice 8. Allowing the Universe to Feel Proud of You

Do Practice 1, Heartfullness Meditation. When you feel your heart is wide open and filled with Source Energy, when your mind feels relaxed and filled with love and your body feels relaxed and filled with your Divinity, ask from your heart, your precious, beautiful heart – ask your Inner Being to let you feel how proud the Universe is of you. As you feel this, allow this feeling to flow into you from every direction. Feel it saturate your heart with that golden, glittering energy. Allow it to drench your mind in the glory of the Entire Universe being proud of you. Allow your body to feel how proud the Universe is of it.

The Entire Universe is always proud of you. There is nothing you can do to stop it from being proud of you. When you start allowing that feeling of being worthy of the Universe's pride in you, when you practice feeling proud of all you have accomplished – even if you have not done anything significant (to you) yet, you will feel yourself feeling better emotionally and physically, and in every way.

Even if you are still in bed as you read this because you are too tired or pained to get up, just allow yourself to recognize that the Universe is proud of you *NOW*. There is nothing you need to do to be worthy of the Entire Universe being proud of you. You are worthy of it now. The more you let it in, the better you will feel.

When you have spent some time, a few days or a few weeks, or however long it takes you, really allowing in the feeling of the Universe being proud of you, till you feel all the empty pockets are all filled with that shining, glowing energy, then start allowing yourself to receive this feeling of being proud of yourself. Once you have practiced being proud of yourself for a few days or weeks or months and you feel solid in it, then share it with those you encounter or think of.

Feel proud of the people in your life. Feel proud of anyone or anything you encounter. Feel proud of your amazing body.

As you do this, you will find your body feeling healthier, more energized. Your body will feel stronger, more secure. More loved. Your relationships will feel richer, sweeter, more connected.

Practice being proud of the easy things and the things that you never thought to be proud of before. As you shift your vibration on each thing, your life will transform more and more. And so will your magical, beautiful, valuable, worthy body.

I feel so proud of you no matter what you have done or where you are or have been.

Feeling the Celebration

I had grown up celebrating the good moments, like most of us did. But that is only part of the story.

I was on the phone with my old phone company and they were telling me about some charge that seemed totally ridiculous. I got off the phone and in that moment I felt angry and I heard myself curse at my sweet, lovable phone company (that I am no longer with).

The minute I heard myself, I realized I was way out of alignment, but then I heard the Universe say, "You are so adorable when you are out of alignment." I felt so surprised. I said, "Are you sure?" And I felt so much love rushing in. Then I felt the sensation that there was a celebration going on all around me. I felt the energy of applause, of a band playing music. I felt the sounds of cheering, I felt the energy of a parade for me… I could not shake it off – nor did I want to. It felt like epic celebration. It felt fantastic. It felt like victory.

I asked my Inner Being about it and the clarity I felt was that everyone and everything is always being celebrated, we are always adorable and adored. Unconditionally. Eternally. Infinitely. That shifted my mind about only celebrating the good things. I wanted to follow the Universe's example.

I felt the Entire Universe is a party of vast celebration for everyone and everything. I felt soooo happy feeling this and I practiced being aware of it over and over and over. Then I practiced *being* that celebration, that party of life. I felt all the cells of my body cell-ebrating. (This always feels like my cells are dancing, and playing with each other inside my body.) I practiced knowing I was adorable no matter what I did.

I celebrated when I was tired. I celebrated my pain. I celebrated my lack of alignment. I celebrated any mistakes. I celebrated my achievements, I celebrated synchronicities, I celebrated everything that came in my path. I felt my cells cell-ebrating more and more. I practiced being unconditional in my celebration. I felt my cells so happy, and it still feels like there is an unconditional party in my body.

As I felt this, I got happier and happier. My energy increased vastly. My pleasure was increasing. My relationships improved. My finances improved… it felt and feels *amazing*. Every time I meditate, I cannot help but feel that celebration. I feel it when I am not meditating too. It's here for us all. Unconditional celebration.

Are you grasping how very, very loved you are? Are you realizing that you do not need to do anything to be given all the celebration you could ever desire and so much more?

Practice 9. Allowing Yourself to Feel Celebrated

Don't wait for something external or out of your control to happen before you allow in all the celebration that the Universe has for you.

Do Practice 1, Heartfullness Meditation, until your heart is wide open and filled with Source Energy, your mind feels relaxed and filled with love, and your body feels relaxed and filled with your Inner Being. Then ask from your heart, your beautiful, open, kind, loving heart – ask your Inner Being to let you feel how the Universe is celebrating you.

If you can, feel the parade, the musicians, the horns blaring for you, the drums causing your whole being to dance and play. Feel the applause, the party, the glory that is here to let you know you are celebrated.

As you feel this, allow this feeling to flow into you from every direction. Feel it drench your heart. Allow this feeling of being celebrated to fill your mind with the magnificence of the Entire Universe celebrating you. Allow your body to feel how much the Universe celebrates you. Allow yourself to recognize that the Entire Universe is celebrating you. Allow the joyful, fun, buoyant energy of being celebrated to drench your whole being. Feel your cells cell-ebrating, feel their joy.

As you practice allowing yourself to feel this over and over, gently start to apply it to every part of yourself. Practice telling your amazing body that you celebrate it, practice telling your mind that you celebrate it.

Once you have been allowing yourself to receive this celebration so that you feel so resourced, so adored, then allow it to flow though you and out to everyone in your path. Celebrate anything and everything you can. Do it like a fun game. Do it because it feels so wonderful to celebrate the good things that you want to come in and to feel that same level of celebration for the unwanted things that come in. Doing this puts you in total power. You will feel more of your invincible nature. And your body *loves* when you feel your invincible nature!

This whole chapter has been about you receiving what you need in order to flow it into yourself and your life.

If you practice receiving first, then you will always be fueled in whatever you do. Loving yourself, loving your life, loving your body, loving others becomes effortless because you receive that love, that approval, that acceptance, that understanding, that pride in you, that celebration *first*, then flowing it to yourself or others is effortless. It is your natural state to be resourced in every way and for life to be effortless and fun. And when you are hooked up to Source Energy, everyone else is off the hook!

This poem came to me while I was making my breakfast, the day I recognized the celebration that was happening all around and in us:

My cells have all become
master musicians
and they have been playing
vibrant music
and throwing wild ecstatic parties
in my body
all day and all night
in celebration
of themselves, me, and each divine moment!
Electric streams inside me are vying for who can
serenade me internally in the most exquisite ways.
I am drinking rainbows
and eating stars
I've dressed myself in sunshine
and perfumed my body with the most fragrant flowers.
Oceans and wild rivers
Are rushing to me,
eager to carry me anywhere
I want to go.
The sky has bent down
and is ravishing me all over with kisses and caresses
inside and outside of my body…
Gosh, it's only 8 a.m.
…Now what?!
By Karen Lorre

Chapter 6

Transforming Easily

A s you have seen in the beginning chapters, we are systematically opening you up to receive so that we can clear your negative painful thoughts that cause pain in the body. Painful thoughts lead to physical pain and fatigue. The more pleasurable thoughts you have, the better your body will feel. I have seen a direct link from feeling emotional pleasure to feeling incredible physical pleasure, hence all this focus on feeling good emotionally. Pleasure is the antidote to pain.

But all of these pleasurable emotions and thoughts must be experienced, not just read about. If you simply read these practices and don't actually do them or do them inconsistently, then they will have little or no effect.

Here is a reminder of the paradox I mentioned before. It feels so tricky, because if you do something because I or someone else suggests you do it, not because you want to do it, not because it feels good to do it, then it really has little effect. The only attitude that works to do things is to do it because it feels wonderful to do, not because I tell you to do it or you think you should do it, but because it feels wonderful to you to do it.

And it feels important to find ways to make any practice that bene-fits you feel wonderful to do!

So, how do you do that?

Well, for me, I discovered that I had been doing this naturally all my life in at least in one area.

I couldn't understand how so many people hated to exercise, but for me exercise is one of my favorite things to do.

I love to exercise. My body loves to exercise. Exercise feels like a treat for me. Exercise feels like a party to me, even when I do it by myself. I always look forward to exercising. It feels so fun to move my body and to exercise. Exercise feels fun. Exercise feels like play-ing… I realized that I had been thinking thoughts like that my whole life. In fact, as I write this book, I take a break about every hour and I exercise. I also have a bike desk, which is a stationary bike with a desk connected to it, so I have been writing this book while riding the bike as well. And it feels wonderful!

As I listened to other's thoughts about exercise, I could hear the difference in the way I naturally thought about exercise.

I know that if I practice any thought enough, I can create a new thought. In fact, at one of Dr. Joe Dispenza's advanced workshops, he showed a time-lapse video of one neuronal structure in the brain and how it had been established there for some time. Then he showed, in fast time-lapse action, how a new neuronal structure was growing as this person whose brain they were filming started thinking a new type of thought.

We watched as the new neuronal structure grew and grew – and as the one that was receiving no attention was simply falling away. In the video this happened over a few minutes; Dr. Joe said that in reality, it happened over a few months of practicing a new thought. The original neuronal structure that had been ignored actually disappeared in the video and the new thought pattern that had been practiced over time was now in its place as a new neuronal structure.

The brain has plasticity. We have the ability to shift and change our thoughts. We have the ability to create new synaptic connections. But the shifts happen with consistent practice. The shifts happen with constant repetition. But for the repetition to be truly effective, it must be done in a state of joy and fun and playfulness.

I felt so excited when I became conscious of all the positive thoughts I had about exercise.

Then I realized it had happened naturally with sugar too.

Here's how that happened naturally for me. I had seen a photo by the genius and loving and brilliant Dr. Bruce Lipton where he showed cells in a Petri dish avoiding the side of the Petri dish where sugar was introduced. The cells were actually moving away from the sugar as fast as they could. I felt so much appreciation for Bruce's photo and for the understanding he gave me that my cells really loved healthy food.

I did nothing to change my diet consciously.

I had been practicing all the things I wrote before in this book that I have shared with you and I was feeling so much love for everyone and everything, that everything looked and still looks beautiful, perfect, sparkly, and sweet. I could and still can feel the sweetness in all that I see. I could feel the sweetness in you, in all people, I could see it in their eyes and feel it in my heart. I could feel the sweetness in the sun and how it shines so brightly and so steadily even when there are clouds. I could feel the sweetness in water that is so nourishing to my healthy body. As I started to feel this, I started tasting the sweetness in vegetables.

I tasted the sweetness in fruits. I felt the sweetness in nuts and in everything I was eating.

Then when I had some kind of normal sugary desert, it tasted far too sweet and heavy and fake for me.

With no effort, I let go of all sugar (except the naturally occurring sugar in whole veggies, etc.). I have not had sugar in over six years, and it has felt effortless. It feels totally easy. If I want a dessert, fresh, in season berries feel and taste delicious to me.

And I make a yummy organic raw cacao drink with purified water, stevia or monk fruit, and coconut oil, all blended in my Vitamix.

Now even kale, celery, spinach and broccoli sprouts taste so sweet to me. Moringa powder tastes sweet...

I now taste the sweetness in everything!

I learned years ago that our taste buds change based on what we are eating. The more sugar you eat, the less sugar you can taste in unsweetened food. The more you eat fresh, organic veggies, nuts, seeds, fruit, and proteins, the less processed food you eat, the more your taste buds find the sweetness in all those foods.

I felt so excited that I could now apply this understanding to every area of my life that I wanted to.

Months before it was time to do my taxes, I started focusing on how much fun doing my taxes is. It feels so good to be organized. It feels so wonderful to feel clear. I feel so happy knowing my tax dollars go in part to the fire department and police department and road builders and schools and the postal people. (Yes, I know our money also goes other places, but I only focus on the places it goes that please me....) I feel so delighted to see all the money that came to me during this time period. It feels so good to see all the things I spent money on and how I am so good at buying the things that thrill me even when I look at just the receipts. I feel so happy to pay my amazing accountant, Carilyn Davidson, for her wonderful help.

As I focused like this, my desire to do my taxes effortlessly increased. After practicing thoughts like that for a few months, my taxes have become fun, easier, and I felt much more clear about them.

This is the practice that you can apply to any area that you want to have more flow.

I do it with food, too. Here's an example about how I created new thoughts about food. I just practiced these thoughts over and over any time I thought of food, and now they are automatic.

"I love eating healthy nourishing, food that makes my body sing with energy and joy. I feel so happy eating lots of fresh organic greens. I feel so much energy eating organic everything. I love eating whole food, food that the earth or its creatures made. I feel so happy eating lots of food that nourishes my body. I feel so good eating like people ate before we had farming, so no grains or processed foods. I feel so good eating broccoli sprouts (they have sooooo many health benefits!!!). And moringa powder (also packed with so much goodness) and all foods that really nourish my beautiful, precious, lovable body."

As I practiced thinking like this, my diet got healthier and healthier and healthier, EFFORTLESSLY.

Practice 10. Upgrade Your Thoughts

You can practice upgrading your thoughts about any area you like. The more you shift your thoughts to be in alignment with all you desire, the easier life will be. Ease is integral to health!

As you go through your day, keep a notepad or use the notes app on your phone to make a note when you recognize negative thoughts on any subject. Then when you have time, write new upgraded thoughts for yourself, and pretend you are an actress or an actor and repeat the new script on that subject until it feels like you own it, it is yours, it is automatic.

The best way to do this is to find a way to feel joyful or deeply relaxed first, then practice repeating the new upgraded thoughts. If you feel like it's work, then stop practicing and go do something that feels good (eat, nap, meditate, write out things you appreciate, exercise, see friends, have sex, be in nature, dance, go for a walk, etc.). Then, as you feel better again, start to practice saying your new upgraded thoughts about your subject.

Only do it for as long as it feels good. Keep repeating this practice of finding a way to feel good, repeating your new script, then when the joy leaves, go back to finding a way that feels good.

As you do this, you are using Hebb's Law with the Law of Attraction. Hebb's Law states, "Neurons that fire together, wire together." You are wiring a good feeling with these upgraded thoughts. And as these neurons of joy and your new upgraded thoughts fire together, you will find both your brain and Law of Attraction helping you to keep your new script active. Do this until you really find these are your automatic thoughts on that subject.

You can do this on the subject of my practices as well, so that you feel desirous of doing these practices (they are all really fun to do naturally, so it's a win-win and may feel super easy for you!).

Bypassing My Personality to See the Best in Me

Transforming Relationships

A lot of people have talked about how important it is to focus on the positive aspects of any person in any relationships you have. That does feel like a valuable and wonderful practice.

In fact, our bodies are a reflection of our thoughts, so when we feel stress or worry or concern about ourselves or another (or about anything), we are actually harming our body and harming the other as well. It does not matter if we feel stress about a politician, a relative, someone in the news, someone you know that is in a challenging time, or even if you feel stress from watching a TV show or movie, or reading a negative book – all of that negative focus harms you, it harms your body and prevents you from helping anyone.

When you feel good emotionally, you are benefitting your body in every way. When you feel good about yourself or another, you are benefitting your body and your life, and you are benefitting them as well.

When I first started to practice trying to feel good about people and finding their positive aspects, I would also activate all the negative aspects that I was not wanting. Just thinking of these people whom I had some resistance about activated that resistance. I did not feel capable of focusing on only their positive aspects. The personality of the other person and my personality got in the way! Giggle.

As I prayed about this, my Inner Being gave me a great awareness. I know that everyone has their own Inner Being. My Inner Being suggested that the more I focus on the all goodness of that person's Inner Being and bypass their personality, the easier it would be. I could skip the personality completely and just tune to their Divine Self. This made writing out positive aspects about others so much easier and more fun.

The first person I did this with was myself. I first wrote out all the aspects of Source Energy that I could. I then practiced ascribing all these aspects to myself. I wrote this every morning by hand for a couple of years.

What happened was amazing. My body kept feeling more and more pleasure. People could feel my alignment more and more. Everywhere I went people said I was glowing, radiant, lit up.

My ability to hear the impulses from my Inner Being increased. My ability to communicate with plants, animals, and those beings now who are non-physical increased. (More about that later.)

All of this amped up my energy substantially. I felt happier and happier and my energy soared. My body felt like it was reverse aging – I still feel like I am getting younger and younger. More and more money flowed (and flows even more now) to me. Opportunities appeared in record speed. And all my relationships got better and better.

This is something that feels so fun to practice. I feel so excited for you as you put this into practice. As you ascribe to yourself any wonderful quality that you desire, you will start to become that more and more. Your body will get healthier. You will feel more energized.

However, remember our paradox: *only do this because it feels good. You are not trying to change anything or make anything happen, you are simply doing a practice that feels wonderful.*

Practice 11. Bypass Your Own Personality to See the Best in You

First, get out a notebook and start writing out all the qualities of Source Energy.

Source Energy is...

Then, look at each of these aspects and ascribe it to yourself.

Use the form, "I am, or I have, or I do, or I feel…"

So for example, my Source Energy is pure, unconditional love. "I am pure, unconditional Love."

Source Energy is infinite loving intelligence. "I am infinite loving intelligence."

Source Energy is bliss. "I feel bliss."

Source Energy is Eternal and Infinite. "I am Eternal and Infinite."

Source Energy is pure fun. "I am pure fun."

Source Energy has love for all. "I have love for all."

Source Energy is abundant in every way. "I feel abundant in every way."

Write this out for yourself.

Find every wonderful quality that you can and that you know is Source Energy and then ascribe it to yourself.

Practice this knowing until it is who you are.

Your body will transform and so will your life. As you do this, you will find old patterns of negative behavior or old negative beliefs about yourself falling away. The happier you feel (authentically happy), the better your body feels. You will feel your energy increase as your self-esteem soars.

Practice 12. Bypass the Personality of Others to See the Best in Them

As I mentioned before, any negative feelings or thoughts you have affect your body in a negative way. Your body is responding to every thought, feeling, and action that you do. When you feel good about all the different areas of your life, your body will thrive more, too. Relationships with others are often a challenge for many. I have found a way for them to feel wonderful, *no matter what the other person does*!

If you have any relationship with anyone that you want to feel better about, this exercise will help. And the more you do it, the better you will feel emotionally, which will cause your body to use its natural genius to bring you the energy and pleasure you are wanting.

If you would feel better, start with Practice 1, Heartfullness Meditation to get into that luscious, loving feeling. You may also want to do Practice 11, Bypass Your Own Personality to See the Best in You, first. Then, when you feel your own divinity, when you feel so wonderful emotionally, when you feel so deeply loved by the Universe, that's when it's best to start this practice.

Do this when you are not with the person you are wanting to focus on. Now apply this to anyone in your life: politicians, parents, partners, children, people you work with, friends – EVERYONE! One by one, begin to ascribe the qualities of their Inner Divinity or Source Energy (whatever you want to call it) to them.

I suggest you start with one person at a time and write out their divine qualities every day until you feel fabulous anytime you think of them, until you can only see their divine qualities, then start with another person.

So for example. Mom's Inner Divinity is unconditional love. "Mom is unconditional love…"

Mom's Inner Divinity is happiness. "Mom is happiness."

Mom's Inner Divinity is divine well-being. "Mom has divine well-being."

Mom's Inner Divinity is eternal well-being. "Mom has eternal well-being."

As I would write this daily, I started to see this in my mom much more easily. The more I saw the Divinity in her, the more I appreciated her and the more she saw it in herself. It became a luscious loop!

Note: ***DO NOT DO THIS TO CHANGE ANYONE!***

The trap that most people fall into when writing positive aspects is that they are trying to change the person about whom they are writing. This tells the Universe that you don't like something about them, which means that those aspects you don't like will come to you more consistently.

Here is the trick: focus on your own divinity and the divinity of others *because it feels good.*

Focus on it to *change the way you feel about them*, not to change them.

Write it so that when you think of that person, or that situation, you feel your heart open and flowing love to them. Write it so that when you think of them, you see them being their best self. Write it so that when you think of them or see them, you feel happy, delighted, free. Write it so you feel excited to see them. That's all this practice is for. It's not to change them, but when you feel good about someone, now you see them more with the eyes of love, and they become free to feel good with you more often. But you can't do it to change them.

For me, when I started to practice this, I wanted to feel better about my ex-husband, but I had a lot of repetitive negative thought patterns about him. Any time I thought of him I would feel my tummy tighten and I would feel my heart racing with fear.

As I sat down to write about him one day, I felt this fear and anxiety and I realized that I was feeling it independent of him. He was nowhere near. I did not know how he was feeling, but I realized that my negative feelings were *my* negative feelings. Not his.

I started to practice focusing on his Source Energy qualities. I wrote out all the wonderful qualities of his Source Energy. I did this almost daily.

On the occasions when we'd see each other, I'd pay attention to my body and if I felt any discomfort, or if I was triggered into negative feelings and thoughts, I realized I had to go back home and write some more of his Divine Qualities.

I could feel that it is never about the person that I think it's about.
It's about my perspective, my thoughts, my feelings about that person.

It's never about the person you think it's about. It's always about your perspective, your thoughts about that person. With my ex-husband it took me about two years (yes, I had some very negative patterns about him that needed to be released!) to feel good around him. I wrote about his divine qualities almost every day and certainly after I saw him if I got triggered. Slowly my whole being and body started to shift. I felt everything in me softening as I practiced this and as old negative patterns flew away.

I felt so happy when one of the times we happened to be in the same circle of friends, I had been actively practicing feeling good while I was there and he came up to me and said, "You're glowing!" That felt like a victory to me. I felt so happy. That was one of the first times he had been kind to me since our divorce. I felt so thankful and it felt wonderful to express my appreciation to him.

But I could feel there was still some resistance within me, so I kept focusing on his divine qualities over and over and over.

I have cleared everything that has come up about my ex-husband now. Now he is free to be whomever he wants to be and I feel total love for him, regardless of what he does. And because of writing his Divine Qualities for so long, I started to see all the amazing things he did in our relationship that I had missed when I was focused on the negative. This filled me with so much appreciation for him, and it also made me much more present to all the goodness others provide for me now as well.

My ex-husband and I actually had a magical, love-filled, adventurous, fun, funny, beautiful, sexy, intuitive, divine, hot, passionate, sweet relationship in many ways! I remember how surprised I felt when I realized what an amazing husband he actually was.

I worked so thoroughly to clear all resistance in me so that I could be totally in love in his presence. And I did. I became an expert on feeling good about anyone unconditionally, mainly because of him. I feel so appreciative of him.

Now we are kind with each other. But more importantly, I feel my heart full and joyful whenever I think of him or see him or hear about him. My love for him has transcended all of his actions and is now so consistent and steady that I feel completely free.

I feel compelled to remind you, *never focus on anyone's divine qualities to change them. Only do it so that you change your perspective, your thoughts, your feelings about them. Let them be who they are and as they are.*

Then get ready to be surprised. (As I wrote that line, I felt a confirmation from my Inner Being in the form of intense orgasmic pleasure. That was my surprise now… what will yours be? Giggle!)

Compassion

Another way people often find themselves triggered into painful thoughts that create pain and fatigue in the body, is that they feel compassion for someone who is suffering. We have often been taught that compassion is feeling the pain of another.

Compassion is a valuable thing. But I define compassion differently than most, and this new definition enables me to have good feelings regardless of whom I am with or of whom I am aware.

I feel so blessed that I was given a beautiful Tibetan painting called a Thankga. It is a painting of the Tibetan Goddess of Compassion, White Tara. It was given to me for my birthday because the person who gave it to me felt how compassionate and kind I am. It was painted by Romio Shrestha, who is the master artist of the Dalai Lama and my friend. Romio said it took him a year to paint it and that it was painted with ground up minerals (ground up gold and silver and lapis and rose quartz, etc.). He told me that he said the mantra for White Tara with every stroke of his brush as he painted her.

Romio had told me to focus on White Tara while I meditated, and he said she would teach me her secrets. For about two years, every morning when I meditated, I would look at her for several minutes before I closed my eyes.

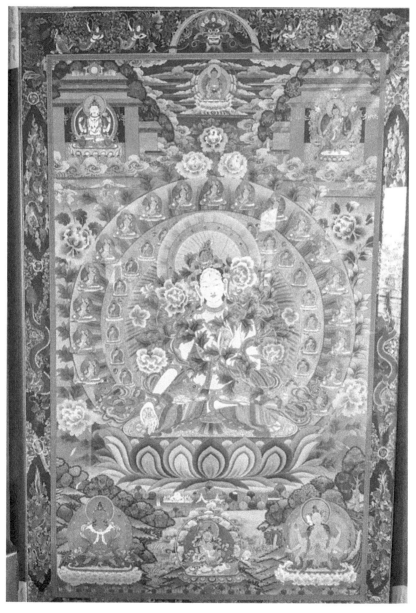

The Tibetan Thankga of the Goddess White Tara, who is the Goddess of Compassion. Painted by Romio Shrestha – the master artist to the Dalai Lama.

What I learned over this time is that this beautiful Goddess of Compassion is in her pure bliss. She has Buddha and flowers all around her. She is connected to her divinity. Her third eye is open and the eyes on her hands and feet are open. She is seeing with the eyes of Source.

And she is shining her bliss out to all below, sending that pure bliss so that the villagers may remember their own bliss. As she is in this bliss, she is fully protected and safe. All the Buddhas and other guardians are all around her and she is totally secure. I took Romio's advice and started to practice that kind of compassion.

So now, when I feel compassion, I feel love, I feel kindness, I feel the goodness, the rightness of the other person or people. I feel their divinity, their power, their capacity to have what they desire. I feel them having the fulfillment of whatever it is they desire. I feel them happy, celebrating, in total joy. I feel them being the pure bliss of who they really are. I feel their infinite intelligence, their brilliance, the tranquility of their Inner Being.

Again, I did this not to change anyone – though people feel amazing with me – I did this because it felt wonderful. I did this so that I would see the best in everyone and so that if they felt inspired to rise up they would see my beacon of confidence in them and it would feel easier for them too.

My life changed. I became tranquil, peaceful no matter what was happening to myself or others. And this affected my body in an amazing way. Just as your body will be affected in a positive way as you put this into practice.

I practiced beaming my bliss everywhere.

My energy increased more, I had no more pain by this time. My life just felt better and better and better.

Now, I define compassion as "Feeling the same as my Inner Being and their Inner Being feels about the subject." So in this case as well, I bypass the personality of the person, animal, plant, or situation and go straight to their source.

My Inner Being knows all is always well. My Inner Being knows that everyone is eternal and infinite (more about that later). My Inner Being knows that anytime anyone has anything that they don't want, their Inner Being is immediately becoming vibrationally what they do want. (I feel thankful to Abraham and Esther Hicks for clarifying this for me. Thank you! I love you!).

This means that the Inner Divinity of all beings is in perfect harmony, joy, bliss, fun, laughter, health, well-being, abundance, freedom, pleasure, power, and love *always*… and so much more.

It feels amazing to tune to the higher vibration of their Inner Divinity while they are in whatever negative state they are in. It feels beautiful to know the perfection of where they are. It feels wonderful knowing that all the challenges I experienced in my past led me to this incredible bliss, this vibrant health and happiness and it feels beautiful to know that this can happen for everyone else too.

It feels sweet to know that any negative emotion anyone is feeling is totally okay, I feel love for them in their negative emotion, and I feel the thrill of what is coming to them.

I don't ask them to change, I simply love them as they are, and I internally feel the thrill of what their Inner Being is embodying.

My compassion 'looks' like regular compassion, but it feels freeing and easy and beautiful. And because I tune to the feeling of their Inner Being, I am siding with what they really want, and that means my Inner Being, their Inner Being, and I are all supporting what they really want. That's three of us all holding the space for the one in pain. This way, I feel certain that they have a much better chance of feeling good and allowing in the fulfillment of their desire than if I drop down into their negative space.

I will hug someone if they are near, I will listen to them, I will nod with understanding at whatever they say and give them the space, the respect, the kindness to be where they are.

And silently, I will feel their well-being, the abundance, the thrill, the health of what they want.

A Real-Life Example of Compassion

One of my dear girlfriends, who happens to be gay, met an amazing man and they had a great spiritual conversation. He asked her for a date. She told him she was gay. He then started to condemn her and tell her God would not love her. He went on and on as he backed away from her.

I felt admiration for my friend, because she was able to be kind and loving to him and not let his anger hurt her. (This is true compassion!)

I watched as many of her other friends condemned this man for condemning her.

I realized it does not matter if it's this man condemning anyone for their sexuality, or if it's others condemning this man for his prejudice – everyone (except for my brilliant friend) was missing the real opportunity for compassion. And that is okay, but there is a way that feels more fun.

I felt how the Universe loves each of us so unconditionally. I saw the divinity, the kindness, the love, the brilliance in my friend. I saw the love, the beauty, the bliss of the man who condemned her. And I saw the perfection, the grace, the divinity of my friend's friends who condemned him. I remained in pure bliss and I beamed it out to all involved.

This provides me with greater health. It provides each of the people involved a chance to feel their own divinity more easily. And it brings peace to the situation. I cannot transmit my love and compassion if I am not feeling it. And the more love, compassion, and bliss I feel, the better my body feels. The more love, compassion, and bliss you feel, the better your body feels.

Another Real-Life Example of Compassion: My Client and Compassion

I was coaching brilliant Elizabeth, who is a well-known professional singer. She was having a hard time with this idea of sending her bliss to someone being unkind. She asked how she could be happy when someone she loved was hurting or having something bad happen to them, or was being unkind to her.

I asked her, "When you sing, if someone in your band sings off-key, do you sing off-key too?"

I saw her eyes light up as she said, "No. In fact, I will make sure I stay on key so that they can hear me and find their way back on."

"Exactly!" I said, "That's exactly like the kind of compassion I use."

Elizabeth's whole body relaxed and she took a deep breath as she let it in, a warm, loving smile spreading across her beautiful face.

Practice 13. Compassion, Feeling the Same as Source

First, make sure you feel lifted up and lightened. Make sure your heart feels wide open and full of love. Then write out what the Inner Divinity in everyone is like. Everyone's Source Energy is always becoming whatever that person, animal, plant, or planet wants in the moment they want it. That means that everyone's Source Energy is full of love, abundant, healthy, having fun, successful at all they do, creative, fully self-expressed, happy, blissful, joyful, free... and so much more. Really let this sink in.

Now apply this to any area of your life about which you want to feel better.

Focus on the gifts that are coming from this experience, situation, or circumstance.

Ask the Source within you if you can feel the same as the Source within you feels about this subject. Write down whatever you perceive that the Source within you feels about that subject. Listen from your heart. I often ask this question, "Inner Being, what do you feel about this situation, person, or circumstance?" then I put my attention on my soft, open heart and listen to the feeling I get.

For me, I get most of my clarity through kinesthetic and emotional knowing, though I also get it audibly and visually and even olfactorily.

You may have audible clarity, visual clarity, emotional clarity, kinesthetic clarity, or olfactory clarity as well, or a combo of them like I do.

As you keep your attention on your soft open heart, allow yourself to feel, or hear, or see, or tune in some way to the higher vibration of the Source within you.

Whatever wisdom comes to you, write it down and put it someplace you can refer to.

Repeat this daily until you see everyone the way that the Source within you sees them. Repeat this until you feel your heart welling up with love no matter who or what you are experiencing.

Again, you are doing this so that you feel good, not to change anyone or any situation or to make anything happen.

But as you do this, as you beam your love and peacefulness and compassionate bliss out to all, then your positive feeling is like a lighthouse beam sending the clear path to all who are ready for it.

They may not follow it in that moment, and that's okay. Let them be where they are. Allow them to find their way when they are ready, not when you are ready for them. Just beam love to them and imagine them as you know they wish to be.

Empathy

Do you ever feel so much empathy that you feel like you are being invaded, or you need to protect yourself? I used to feel like I was so sensitive that I was feeling other people's negative feelings, even those they were not conscious of. I could feel people "invading me" with their negative emotions. I could feel people's anger or fear… it felt like I was carrying so many other people's energies around in me and I was constantly trying to protect myself from these negative energies.

I was home alone one day, and I started to feel some negative energy that seemed to be coming from a friend. I felt frustrated and afraid. "How do I stop this negative invasion?" I asked. I felt inspired to soften my heart. Then I felt a new clarity flow in. I got this clear insight: *If I was feeling negative emotions, it's in me, it's not coming from someone else.*

I can only feel the emotions that are on the same frequency that I am on.

I felt my dear love, Johnny (he is and was nonphysical, but he communicates with me all the time – more on that in a later chapter) telling me when I was twenty-three years old that there were two radio stations I could tune to emotionally: Radio K-LACK or Radio K-LOVE.

I realized I had been tuned to Radio K-LACK. I saw a clear image of my Source Energy beaming me a signal of love, but I had been on the other station, so I was tuning to what I thought were the negative emotions of people who weren't even with me.

I felt so clearly that if I was in a state of love, I would only feel the love from others.

In that moment, I felt like a world of negative energy simply fell away from me. I could breathe deeper. My body felt more supple, more at ease. I physically felt lighter, more free.

I felt a deep breath of fresh air flowing in as I realized that I am the world. If I take care of any negative emotion within me, the whole world will benefit. And I felt this new truth:

> *I want to have empathy with Source Energy, I want to be sensitive to Source Energy. Just as I want to feel compassion with Source, my empathy, my sensitivity wants to be attuned to Source Energy. I realized that my sensitivity is a true gift when I turn it toward my Source Energy.*

I immediately felt a new sense of freedom, confidence, and connection that let me know that this was a relevant thought. I felt lifted up and lightened. I felt clear that I did not need to protect myself from negative energies anymore… love keeps me totally secure.

I felt all that energy I had spent on protecting myself just dropping off me. I realized that whatever I am protecting myself against, I am drawing to me.

All the energy I spent in trying to protect myself from other people's negative energy came back to me. I felt totally enlivened in a new way. My energy skyrocketed. I felt free. My physical energy got stronger and more vibrant as I made a deeper commitment to having empathy and compassion with Source.

Now, I use my sensitivity to feel into what is coming for me and others. And I am amazingly accurate. I use my sensitivity to intuitively say the right thing in the right way to the right people at the right time. My sensitivity, my empathy with Source, puts me in the flow. I feel so attuned to the soothing, loving energy of Source that now I can often just ask a question and the answer flows in.

Most times, I don't even need to ask. I feel completely guided and inspired. This causes me to save so much time, which gives me much more energy and pleasure.

The happier your thoughts, the happier and healthier your body is.

You can have the liberation of all that protective energy, of the pain of being very sensitive, returned to you in the form of more vibrant, youthful, fun, pleasurable energy. And your sense of security will soar.

Practice 14. Empathy with Source

Really allow yourself to meditate on this, knowing that your empathy, your sensitivity is a divine gift when you are using it to attune to Source Energy.

Recognize that any negative emotions that you feel are simply an indication that you let your vibration drop, so you are picking up energies that are irrelevant and don't lift you up and lighten you – so they obviously are not Truth.

Thoughts cannot be the truth if they don't lift you up and lighten you.

Take full responsibility for anything you feel. If you feel it, know it's coming from you and know that you can change your own emotions. Taking responsibility is where the real freedom lives.

Know that Source Energy is pure love and that as you tune to that you are completely safe and secure and you are benefitting the world by being a happier, more love-filled person. Even if you are home alone, if you are feeling happy, feeling loved and loving, then you are a positive force in the world. Being in a state of love in itself is an act of bountiful service.

Recognize that you are the world, and if you take care of your negative emotions, you will benefit the whole world. As Gandhi said, "Be the change that you wish to see in the world."

Changing Your History

So many of us have had negative experiences in the past that still cause us stress or negative emotion. The better you feel emotionally, the better your body feels.

One Tuesday, I was early to my favorite dancing, singing yoga class, so I sat outside in the courtyard having some tomato basil soup while I waited for the class doors to open. I was thinking of how we can be visioning about the present, visioning about the future, or visioning about the past, and as long as it all felt good in this moment, it was good for us.

Then I thought about how whatever desires I have had, they have all come true *vibrationally*. That's the truth for all of us. Anytime anyone has a desire, their Inner Divinity becomes that which they desire.

I thought of that word, "History." "His Story." Then I changed it in my mind to "Hi Story" – a history that makes me high! As I was feeling this new clarity, I thought about my life.

In real life, I had been a gymnast as a teen, and I had loved it. I still do acrobatics and I love to do handstands and cartwheels and other fun things. The college I went to did not have a gymnastics team, so my only training had been while I was in high school and at Cathy Rigby gymnastics camp one summer as a young teen. I had wanted to keep growing as a gymnast but there was no opportunity.

In that moment of thinking about how I had been a gymnast with the desire to keep growing in it, I felt this vision flow in.

Suddenly, I felt elated as I saw that I was in the Olympics. I was doing the floor routine. I could see that my form was fantastic, my tricks were high and beautiful, and I could see my vibrant smile. I could feel my body flipping and twisting and feeling so strong and energized. I could hear the joyful music... it felt so fun. I heard the announcers saying, "Look at Karen, she is on it. She is flying through her routine with total grace. Look at her precision, her strength – the crowd loves her." I could hear the crowd chanting and clapping, "Karen! Karen! Karen!" (Hey, this was *my* vision! Giggle!)

I completed the routine and saluted the judges. My big Russian coach picked me up and hugged me while he walked, saying, "Karen, Karen, that was incredible. I am so proud of you!" I could feel my teammates hugging me, congratulating me, so happy for me. I felt so full of love for them. I felt so thankful.

In this vision, all the judges from all the countries stood up, their eyes filled with tears, big smiles on their faces. as they clapped for me. I felt elated as we saw I had the highest score. (Visions don't have to be realistic, they just have to feel good now!)

The scene morphed and I was now on the dais with the gold medal around my neck. I could feel the weight of the medal around my neck. The American flag was held high. The Silver and Bronze winners were next to me with their countries' flags above them. I felt so much love for them.

I felt the bright lights shining at me, so it was hard to see the audience, but I could feel my family and friends directly across from me, cheering me on. As the American anthem was being played, I started to cry. I felt so thankful.

As my tears of appreciation flowed down my cheeks in the courtyard outside my yoga class, I realized that even though I had never made it to the Olympics to compete in real life, my Inner Being had held this vision, this knowing of what I really wanted, and I was receiving it in that moment vibrationally.

I felt profound appreciation for my Inner Being, and I started practicing the thought that I was a gold medal winning gymnast. I know I am not a gold medal gymnast in real life, but it felt so good to feel that I was that gold medal winning gymnast vibrationally. I kept repeating it to myself and remembering the feeling of this amazing vision that had flowed to me.

My yoga class doors opened and as I kept repeating silently, 'I am a gold medal winning gymnast!!' my energy grew and grew and was off the charts. I was doing eight to ten clapping push-ups between each vinyasa. My legs felt stronger. My endurance felt amazing. My balance was solid. Everything I did felt easier than it had ever felt before. I felt more flexible. I felt epically strong. It felt so easy because *yoga is nothing compared to gymnastics…*

After class, my friends said things like, "Wow, Karen, your energy is off the charts tonight! What's going on?"

I simply smiled, "Oh that feels wonderful, thank you, I guess I just feel good…"

But inside I was squealing and clapping, "I am a gold medal winning gymnast!"

As I repeated, "I am a gold medal winning gymnast!" over and over the next few days and weeks, my confidence increased (after all, once you've won a gold medal, you have the knowledge you can do anything!).

My posture got better because I could feel my gymnastic body. My energy increased and I started to work out more and more. My belly got the six-pack abs again. Everything in me got stronger and more fit and toned.

When I went back to that yoga class the following weeks, my energy increased every week I went. The teenagers in class would ask me how I had so much energy. Every week people came up to me and asked why I was so elated, so enlivened. So many people in class said I had the energy of a three-year-old, or a seven-year-old. One lovely lady said I had the energy of a group of happy three-year-olds!

As I kept playing with that thought that I was a gold medal winning gymnast, that I have always been a gold medal winning gymnast, I also realized that all my desires in life had come true:

I realized that I have always been in alignment, I have always been healthy. I have always been pure love. I have always been kind. I have always been beautiful, I have always been abundant... it felt so wonderful to feel into this that I kept repeating those phrases and others. I have always been aligned. I have always been healthy, I have always been wise...

I was just doing this silently in my head, but I felt amazed when I realized that the whole world was listening.

Within a few days I started to receive communications from people I had not talked to in twenty or more years. One man said, "Karen, I installed your TV when you lived in NYC and I always remembered how kind and loving you are."

I had not lived in NYC for over twenty-five years at that time. It felt so sweet that he remembered me. Then another girl said that I had helped her twenty-eight years before by giving her some guidance that she was still using and every time she did it she thought of me with appreciation. She said she appreciated how loving and kind I was back then. Then others kept telling me the same sorts of things: "Karen, you've always been loving. You've always been so wise. You've always been so fun..."

And I realized more deeply that *the whole Universe is always listening.*

Because I changed my history with that vision of being a gold medal winning gymnast, making it a Hi Story that took me higher, and because I changed it with that further understanding that I have always been all the love and health and pleasure and kindness and wisdom and abundance that I wanted, I felt better and better in my present so of course, my present changed, which changed my future and my body.

Today my body feels so energized, so healthy, so fit, I have had the awareness that I have been a gold medal winning gymnast for the last five years as of this writing and my desire to work out has increased exponentially.

Here's another more private bit of a Hi Story that shifted for me.

I was lying in bed, still very relaxed, after just waking up, thinking about sexual pleasure, when a vision flowed in.

I saw myself as a little girl, in my bedroom in the afternoon, playing with my body sexually. In this vision, my enlightened mom came into my bedroom, saw what I was doing, and said to me, "Oh Karen, I feel so delighted you have found the pleasure in your body! I feel so proud of you. Your sexual pleasure is innocent and beautiful. Do you know that if you have orgasms every day, it is a benefit to your whole body and brain? You should play with yourself every day! And Karen, there are so many wonderful sensations you can have all over your body. Explore every part of your body and you will find so much pleasure."

My envisioned mom kissed me on the forehead and walked out, closing the door so I would be in peace and solitude. I felt so safe, so loved, so understood.

In the vision, when I came out of my bedroom, my mom and dad were there and my dad had brought me flowers. He gave me a big hug and said, "Your mom told me that you found your sexual pleasure and I feel so proud of you. Your sexual pleasure is so innocent, pure, beautiful, and healthy and should be celebrated. The more you give yourself sexual pleasure, the happier and healthier you will be."

He gave me the large bouquet of flowers, which smelled so fragrant, and a hug. I felt like the most loved, cherished, fortunate little girl in the world. As I envisioned this, again I was crying with this new clarity and with deep appreciation.

I could feel my body relaxing on a deep level. I could feel the energy of my sexual organs feeling sweeter.

I felt some new thoughts flow from this vision: "My sexuality has always been supported. I have always been sexually safe. Feeling pleasure is good for my health and my well-being. My body has always been pleasured. My parents are amazing. I feel so thankful for my parents. I feel cherished. My sexuality is cherished. I feel treasured. I feel so feminine. I feel safe to be feminine…"

These new thoughts felt so fun to practice.

I replayed that vision over and over, and my relationship with my body improved. My body has become so full of pleasure that it's amazing. I feel incredible pleasure in the most subtle areas, like my knees, or along my spine, or on my cheek…

My relationship with my parents improved; my ability to feel pleasure increased. And I started to attract healthier, more sensuous men as well. (That's a whole other book!)

Because I have had these visions and many others that have rewritten my past, I now can see all the real-life goodness that was already there for me that in previous times I had missed. I started to see so many bright spots in my life that my whole life seemed to shift into a happier past, which lead to a happier present. I felt like my whole past was supporting me, fueling me, loving me. Now I only see the goodness, the happy times, the healthy times in my past. My whole life feels like epic love.

Practice 15. Creating Your Hi Stories

The more you find the Hi Stories in your History, the more your body will thrive. Each time you do this on any past experience, you will uncover a fountain of energy and well-being that will source you in new ways.

First, get into a happy, open hearted, love-filled state. Then, think about any desires you have had in your past that seemed like they never came true and start to imagine them as if they had come true. See them in every detail with visual, audio, fragrances, physical sensations, tastes, and emotions. Let the whole new Hi Story fill in.

Do one Hi Story at a time.

Once you have this new vision, you can write it down and then read it or envision it over and over. Again, this must be a vision that feels good to think about now. It does not have to be realistic, it just has to feel good.

You are not doing this to change anything, you are simply doing this to feel good in this moment.

The more you practice feeling and experiencing and telling this new Hi Story, this story about your past that makes you feel higher, the more you will feel new energy, new pleasure flowing in. Simply practice the new awareness consistently until you feel it has become true for you.

Only practice it to feel good right now. If you get new good feeling thoughts because of this new Hi Story, write them down and practice them as well.

You can do this on every part of your life.

And when you feel good about your past, your past fuels this moment, so your present feels more fun, which causes your future to be even brighter! And as you feel better and better, your body will respond with more and more pleasure and energy. YAY YOU!

Read this poem as if you are bringing this into your own experience:

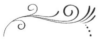

This morning the sky bent down and kissed my feet
Exclaiming to all who would listen the glory of my being
The trees joined in, their resplendent leaves glistening,
dancing with joy, knowing of the bliss that resides in
everything.
The light of the stars and the sun chimed in,
entwining around me like rapturous lovers in wild embrace
My cupboards reach out to me, softly, tenderly letting me
know that they too hold the secret of the Universe

*The secret that is so obvious we CANNOT NOT shout it
from every cloud, every sunbeam.
The secret every newborn baby is beaming with its eyes –
before it's been trained to forget.
My heart grows wider than all of creation, and I feel the
love in everything and everyone.
I dissolve into a wave of ecstasy
that flows in me and around me,
carrying me on the momentum of love.
This Universe is having its way with me!
The sun, the moon, and the stars
have been peeking in my heart,
uncovering my every wish
and rounding up the trees and flowers and birds and sky
to gather
all I desire from every corner of the earth
and bring it to me in the most delicious ways,
like I am the cherished one of the Universe.
But I know the truth:
We are all the cherished ones of the Universe!
The sky is bowing to your feet,
exclaiming your glory
Will you join me in this ecstatic party
celebrating
the love
and the
magnificent splendor
that you are?*
By Karen Lorre

Chapter 7:

Changing Cultural Hypnotic Suggestions

Releasing the Cultural Hypnosis

When I was a teen, I had a practice that seemed to open up my mind. I would go to the park, sit under the same tree every time, and just allow the tree to sort of talk to me, to inspire me. I didn't know what meditation was, but I was doing a rudimentary form of it, because I was in a deep listening mode while I was with that wonderful tree.

As I practiced connecting with that tree, more and more clarity came to me.

I was in my AP science class in high school one day when I felt a new clarity.

My teacher was talking about how there are trillions of germs everywhere, on each desk, on every doorknob, on our pens or pencils... pretty much everywhere we touched.

In that moment, I realized that the only time I ever got a cold or any bacterial or viral sickness was not when I was around people who were sick, because lots of times I had been around people who were sick, and I had been hugging them, kissing them, and I remained fine.

I realized I only got sick when I had been stressed, which lowered my immune system.

A metaphor came to me. You know those tennis ball machines, that shoot the ball at you from the opposite side of the court and then you hit the ball back? I had this vision of the tennis ball machine spewing out balls of bacteria and germs and viruses, and if you were relaxed and agile, if you were on your game, you would hit the balls back to the other side of the court and be healthy and strong and vibrant.

Then I imagined that if you were distracted, or stressed or not playing well, you would miss a lot of the balls filled with bacteria, germs, and viruses that the machine sent to you. Your court would be filled with missed balls, which would make it more likely that you would trip and be more susceptible to the viruses, bacteria, and germs that were present in your court.

That felt like the perfect metaphor for me to understand how I had gotten sick and how not to get sick in the future.

When I felt that clarity, it felt like this new power woke up within me.

I had heard the commercials about it being 'cold and flu season' and I knew in that moment that that did not apply to me, nor to you unless you believe it. I realized it was our belief about our vulnerability and stress that was making us sick, not the season we were in.

I could feel it was what I called at the time – and still do – 'Cultural Hypnotic Suggestions.'

I realized that those commercials and commercials like that were actually programing us to get sick in those times.

In that moment, I felt certain I wanted to clear all Cultural Hypnotic Suggestions from myself. And I felt clear that listening to some commercials and watching some TV shows that were full of negative cultural hypnotic suggestions was not something I wanted to do much of. I saw it had been programming me in ways that were not good for me. I did not want to be programmed with someone else's agenda. I did not want cultural hypnotic suggestions imprinted upon me. I don't want you to be full of cultural hypnotic belief systems, either!

That belief that someone else can make me sick was the first one to go. I experimented with this and found that I could be around people when they had bronchitis, or the flu or whatever, and I could kiss them, hug them, and support them in feeling better, and if I was relaxed and loving, if I had no stress, I did not get sick.

I also saw that the few times I have gotten a cold or a flu, it was always when I had been stressed or was not listening to what my body wanted. It was my stress or not listening to what my body was wanting that got me sick, not the bacteria, virus, or anything else. I have practiced this for most of my adult life and I now have no fear of germs or of anyone being sick around me because I feel utterly relaxed, so I feel invincible. I'm so happy and I feel my immune system is totally happy too and totally able to handle any germs, bacteria, or viruses or anything that comes my way, precisely because I am so relaxed.

You can do this too. As you start to release negative programming from your culture, you can recognize the power and well-being your body has and its ability to deal with the trillion plus germs, viruses and bacteria that are always around you, easily, when you are relaxed and feeling good.

And I feel the same way about the weather. I would always hear, "It's cold out, wear a sweater or you'll get sick."

It never made any sense to me that cold weather could make you sick – unless you were stressed about something and then your immune system would be down, and you would get sick.

I had been wearing sweaters so I would not get sick when I felt so clearly that my feeling wary of the cold weather was what was making me sick. My fear of getting sick was making me sick. I stopped worrying about what the weather was like and dressed how I wanted, and I just trusted I would be healthy and that is exactly what has happened. It does not matter if I am in extreme heat, extreme cold, or anything in between. If I feel healthy emotionally, if I feel confident and I am not guarding against anything but instead I am relaxed, listening to my body, and welcoming whatever comes, I stay healthy in all weather.

I just got back from the high arctic where we swam in four-degree Celsius icy arctic ocean water. I felt so exhilarated and happy swimming in that water. I knew it would make me healthier, not sicker. And indeed, I felt incredibly healthy after and have remained so. Whatever we guard against we draw to us.

Practice 16. Release Any Cultural Hypnotic Suggestions That Don't Serve You

When we believe in things that are not true, or that are negative, they can harm our bodies and make us more susceptible to *everything*. The more you release negative cultural hypnotic suggestions, the better your body will feel, the more energy you will have, and the more pleasure you will have.

Become aware of any cultural hypnotic suggestions you have bought into and decide what *you* choose to believe. You are in charge of you and your world, not society, not the news, not advertisers, not doctors, not your parents, not your children, not your teachers…

Once you determine what you want to practice believing, then practice it until you own it, until it's impossible for you to think the way you were trained. Practice so that you feel wonderful emotionally when you think of it. You will tap into your deep and profound strength in a new way.

Letting Go of Guarding

Whenever we guard against anyone or anything, we are actually drawing it to us. Being wary or afraid or protective against getting sick actually makes us more likely to get sick. Being wary or protective or defensive against experiencing anything actually brings it to us. The only state that renders us totally secure is in that state of pure love, pure invincibility, pure joy. All protection, defense, wariness, and fear weakens you and your amazing, genius body.

Practice 17: Release Any Guarding or Protection

As I mentioned above, any guarding or defensiveness or trying to protect yourself or your body, or anything is actually harming you. It causes tension and stress and you become less able to deal with the things that come your way. The better you feel emotionally, the more your body will thrive.

Pay attention to any areas where you are guarding, protecting, or defending yourself or another. Pay attention when you are justifying or rationalizing something. It may feel like tension in your body. It may feel like a tightness that wants to be released. All these emotional states bring you what you don't want. When you are relaxed, you will allow in what you do want.

When you find any of the above tensions, breathe into wherever that protective energy is in your body and let it go. Feel it disappear, dissolve. Practice feeling that relaxed confidence of health and well-being in any situation. The more you keep your heart full of love, soft and open, the more you feel that tranquility of letting your heart lead, the more you will discern any tensions, guarding justification, or protections. As you discern them, you will feel the stress that they cause, which you can consciously learn to relax your body around so that you can be soft with it.

I do a type of deep relaxation, like hypnosis, that enables me to rewrite negative patterns easily. I do this with myself and my clients. The more you learn to relax your body, the more receptive to new ideas you will be. Deep relaxation also makes it easier for you to feel the Divine Inspirations that are always coming to you. (More on that later!)

Releasing the Cultural Hypnosis of Dieting

Thinking Thin

When I was in high school, I came home from running around the park the day after Christmas and asked my mom where the large box of chocolates we had received were.

My mom shrugged, "Oh, I ate them all."

It was only 1 p.m. "What? You ate them all? You are going to get so fat!"

"No I won't," she smiled.

"Why not?" I felt so curious!

She shrugged again. "I think thin…" Then she smiled and walked away.

I felt amazed. I felt compelled to ponder that sentence, "I think thin," for the next several years. As the years passed, I realized I was feeling so many healthy inspirations that kept my body in the same athletic shape as it was in high school. I realized that having a great body did not have as much to do with what I did, but it had everything to do with how I felt about it.

And then that feeling of knowing I will be thin always, inspired positive actions in alignment with what I wanted. My body still looks about the same as it did when I was a competing gymnast in high school.

What does thinking thin mean?

I never have counted calories. If I am hungry, I eat, if I am almost full, I stop eating. I told my body my skin would always be smooth and soft and it still is. I feel inspired to work out and stretch daily. I feel compelled to eat tons of healthy vegetables, nothing processed and everything from nature. I never worry if something will make me fat – in fact, I eat a ton of healthy fat every day. I listen to what my body wants.

The other night I went to a vegan restaurant and I got a kohlrabi salad with watercress and a side of brussels sprouts. The brussels sprouts were so yummy that I had a second plate and then a third plate. I felt full after the third plate! Giggle. But I listened to my body and that's what it felt it wanted, so I trusted it.

I also eat super slowly and chew my food well so it's liquified before I swallow it, so that my body can easily feel when it's getting full.

I suggest that you start enjoying eating whole food that the earth has grown, food that is unprocessed, like lots of vegetables, nuts, seeds, fruit, and proteins. I suggest that you chew your food slowly, so it becomes liquified before you swallow it.

I learned when I was a teenager, that there is about a twenty-minute lag time between the stomach and the part of the brain that registers fullness. I eat slowly (I eat slowly because I love food and I love the taste and want to savor it!) and because of that my mouth can alert my stomach on how to digest the food optimally, and my stomach can alert my brain and I will know to stop when I feel almost satiated and not after. If my body craves a certain healthy food, I follow that (hence the three orders of brussels sprouts!).

And I listen to my body. If a food makes me tired, I stop eating it. If a food gives me healthy energy, I eat it more often. I eat to fuel my body with energy. I also eat everything in a state of love. *I feel vibrant energy eating only foods that nourish my body.* I have nothing that is not good for me in my diet. By listening to my body, I have easily let go of eating grains, sugar, caffeine, and most dairy. This has made my body feel so steady in energy all day long.

The more you eat lots of fresh unprocessed vegetables, and other whole foods, the more you chew your food, the more you eat to fuel your body with nourishing food, the better you will feel. *The more you feel happy and in love when you eat, the more you will be guided to the food that is right for you.* Pay attention to food that makes you tired and gently let it go.

I suggest you don't judge any foods in a negative way as that will create more stress; instead, love all food, but eat the food that really nourishes your body. More about that next.

Releasing the Cultural Hypnosis of Food Allergies

I know I was not born with any food allergies; all of mine developed. If you decide to try the advice in this section, please check with your trusted health advisor first, since I have only done this with myself and the clients that had allergies develop after they had been on the planet in that body for a while. Always be safe!

When I was about twenty-three, I had been told that I had some food allergies. I avoided those foods so I did not get the nausea that I would get any time I ate them, even when I did not know they were part of the food. I had been sent to the hospital twice with nausea that would not stop for hours after eating those foods.

As I was writing out appreciation one morning, I felt myself become aware of one of the foods to which I had been diagnosed as allergic. I felt nauseous just thinking of that food. And yet, that food was nowhere around me. I felt myself become aware that the nausea I felt had nothing to do with the food. It had everything to do with my *thoughts* and *feelings* about the food.

In that moment, I felt determined to experiment with loving that food unconditionally. I practiced loving it for about three months. Every time I wrote out appreciation (which is most mornings), I would appreciate anything I could about it.

I practiced thinking about that food and loving it and I got so that I felt confident that I could love it unconditionally.

I wrote this not to make anything happen, but just so I would feel good when I thought about that food.

After around four months of this practice, I was out to eat at a great restaurant, and I ordered some food but had not read the fine print that said that the food I was supposedly allergic to was in that dish. I ate it and realized that food was in there. I relaxed and paid attention to how I felt. I felt inspired to finish that dish. My body felt completely fine. There was no sign that I had had any allergy to that food at all. My energy felt high. I felt elated. Now I eat that food whenever I want, and I always feel awesome when I do.

I felt so clear that I had had that negative reaction to that food because at some time in the past I had eaten it when I had resistance or stress. Because I had been in resistance, my body could not process the food in the right way. Then it had a bad reaction to that food.

I had thought it was about the food. But it was about my thoughts *and* feelings *about the food.*

I systematically practiced loving each food I wanted to eat. Now I only eat in a place of pure love and my body digests everything perfectly.

Our bodies are a reflection of our thoughts, not just the thoughts about our bodies. That's why we are examining so many areas of life – so that you can feel better in every area of life.

The more that you love your body and your metabolism and the food you eat, the more you love the food you don't eat, the more you are in a state of love, the better your body will feel.

Again, you can practice loving a food, feeling good about a food, but never eating it if it is not right for you. Even just loving the food will benefit your body!

Practice 18: Releasing Any Cultural Hypnosis of Food

Become aware of what your belief system is about food or eating. If your thoughts are thoughts that feel good, you don't need to do anything.

If your thoughts could feel a lot better, then start to design your own beliefs about that subject, whether it is food, or any area.

Become aware if you tell yourself things like, "Any time I eat that food, I get sick!" or "Oh, just smelling food causes me to gain weight!"

or, "No matter what I do I can't lose weight." or any other negative programs you have been running.

Once you become aware of them, create a new, empowered way to think.

For example, "My body digests all my food perfectly and I have the perfect metabolism."

Or, "My body loves to be at the perfect weight for me."

"It's so easy for me to be the perfect weight for me!"

"My body loves me!"

"My body loves to be healthy, fit and strong."

These upgraded thoughts, or your own, need to be practiced, repeated, over and over and over until they feel true. Until you own them. Until they are yours. Create new upgraded thoughts and repeat them until you feel them being repeated back to you by your very cooperative brain. When it becomes automatic that you feel awesome when you think about your body or your metabolism or that food or substance, that's when you get the real benefit to your beautiful, precious, *amazing* body!

Case History:

My client had an allergy to horses and hay. As we worked together and I relaxed her deeply, we discovered that when she was little, her brother had been unexpectedly and severely injured. She was told this when she was out taking care of the family horses.

The shock, the fear, the uncertainty of what would happen to her brother and her parents, who were very scared and stressed at the time, scared her so much. She was crying and crying – still with those horses as she felt this.

As she grew up, she didn't really remember that day. But her body remembered all that stress and resistance when she was around the horses and the hay. So every time she went near any horse or hay or a farm, she would get terrible hives, congestion, and sneezing.

I relaxed her deeply, then we cleared the negative energy of that day her brother had been injured (he recovered fully), so that when she looked back on it she felt peaceful, relaxed, and easy. She practiced feeling that peacefulness and ease while thinking of her brother, and horses and looking at pictures of them and of hay until she felt happy and relaxed while thinking of them.

Her allergies totally disappeared. Now she and her husband have their own horses and she rides almost every day. The freedom she feels looks beautiful on her!

It was not about the horses and the hay. It was about her *thoughts* and *feelings* when she had had that trauma and she had associated it with the horses and the hay.

You can do the same thing. Practice loving everything. Upgrade your history so that any negative experiences are now nourishing to you. Your body will become more and more energized and full of pleasure as you do this.

Practice 19. Releasing Negative Emotions That Caused Allergies

Definitely check with your doctor to see if you should even try this. If you do try it:

Notice how your body feels when you think of that thing to which you are allergic, when you are not near it. Realize that it is probably not that thing but your *thoughts* and *feelings* either about that thing or about some other experience in your life associated with that substance. Experiment: practice finding all the things you appreciate about it whenever you think about it.

Do not engage with that substance or thing until you feel totally peaceful, appreciative, and relaxed when you think of it.

(It may take a few months of practice – unless you can also find the inciting incident when it happened and release all the negative emotions around that incident.)

Once you have the consistent feeling of appreciation, peace, and relaxation when you think of it, then, if you feel inspired to try this and if your doctor agrees, gently expose yourself to it in a very small, safe way.

Expose yourself in a small dose so you can see how your body reacts. Don't be afraid of how your body will react; instead feel your love, your bliss as you try a very small amount.

We draw to us what we fear, so love is the only path.

If your body still has any negative reaction, step back from it and go back to appreciating it every day until you feel total love and adoration for it.

Then again, check with your doctor, and if you feel inspired, try it again in a very small, safe dose. It's not really about eating the food you were allergic to, or exposing yourself to the substance, it's about feeling love and calm and peace around anything. You never need to eat that food or be around the thing you were allergic to; if you feel love when you think about them, you will already be helping your amazing body thrive more.

There may be some things that are not worth bringing back into your life, and it may feel easier to just avoid them. That is good too, but your life will be benefitted by you learning to love them even if you never have contact with them again.

For example, since I was a bio-science major in college and have always been interested in the science of health, I studied so many things throughout my life that talked about how bad sugar and flour and grains are for the body. That's not why I don't eat them. I don't eat them now because they simply fell away from me when I felt all the sweetness and goodness of this world. It just feels good to eat whole foods without any extra sugar or processed grains now. But I still practiced loving sugar and loving grains. I just don't want them in my diet. But I love them. I feel that they are wonderful. That way I feel in alignment about every aspect of food, and I make my choices based on what gives me the most clean, pure, happy feeling.

You never have to eat or be exposed to any allergen, but if you practice loving it when you are not around it, and you get so solid in your love, then you will be aiding your incredible, brilliant body in every way.

Releasing the Cultural Hypnosis of Aging

Our bodies are always responding to what we think, feel, and do. If you are feeling or saying that you feel old, or tired, or achy, then your body is listening to that and recreating that for you. The better you feel emotionally, the better your energy and your pleasure will be.

When I was a little girl, I heard lots of adults say things like, "Now that I am older, I don't do this sport anymore." "Now that I am older, I need at least two cups of coffee to start my day." "Now that I am over thirty, I gain weight so quickly." "I am too old to climb a tree now."

I became aware of these thoughts when I was about twelve. And I vowed to myself that I would never stop climbing trees, never smoke, never drink coffee, and never get old.

I did try drinking coffee for a few years, but I have not had it in over fourteen years and I have no desire to have it anymore. I feel vibrant, amazing energy from the moment I wake up. Coffee now would only make my body more tired. But I feel love for coffee, if you like it. I love coffee, but I choose not to have it in my body.

I still climb trees and anything else I can climb that looks fun. I have never smoked. and I feel younger now than I ever did before.

After hearing all those adults complain about aging, I knew that I would never talk that way. I could hear how they were programming themselves to be old! That horrified me as a young teen. I vowed to myself to program myself better. I started to tell my body it would always be young. I would always play and have fun. I would always feel youthful.

Now that I have been in a state of love and clarity for over a decade as of this writing, I have expanded on this. I feel so clear that we are all infinite, eternal beings. I feel certain that my Inner Being does not age. In fact, I feel so delighted that my Inner Being gets better and better every day in every way.

With every desire I have, my Inner Being becomes the fulfillment of it. The more aligned with my Inner Being I am, the more I, too, get better every day in every way. My body still looks like it did when I was an athletic teenager (without the baby fat). I feel flexible, supple, strong, and youthful. I feel happy in the knowing that I do not need to buy into the cultural hypnosis that I have to age. In fact, most of my body has felt younger and younger.

I used to wear glasses to read, then I tuned back into this great knowing that I could stay youthful, and the more I was seeing the world from the eyes of love, the better my eyesight got. My eye doctor used to say in surprise as he tested my eyes, "Your eyes are reverse aging!" I stopped wearing my glasses and I only use them maybe once a month to read something really small. My functional medicine doc (he's my friend!) told me that I have the physiology of a seventeen-year-old. That's what happens when I practice feeling ageless, eternal, and youthful! It feels amazing telling my body that it is seventeen years old and watching it looking and feeling better and better!

Practice 20. Releasing the Cultural Hypnosis of Aging

You can tap into your eternal youthfulness easily.

Do Practice 1, Heartfullness Meditation, and feel your heart open, your mind relax, and your body relax.

In that relaxed state, recognize your eternal, infinite, ageless spirit.

Start telling yourself that you are the age you wish to be. (I tell my body and myself every day, many times a day, that I am seventeen – and I hear so many people tell me that my body looks like I am seventeen! I have more energy than most seventeen-year-olds I know, too.) I am not afraid of aging. I love my age. I just feel excited to program my body the way I want it to be.

Tell yourself that you can do and be and have anything you want.

You can tell yourself that you can do any activity and still not do it, and that's what I suggest. I suggest you wait to do any activities that you used to do or that you want to do, until you feel compelled to do them because your body just feels so youthful and amazing. Only do the activities if it feels fun, easy, and you feel totally, one hundred percent confident. Even if you don't do the activities, telling yourself you can do it, telling yourself that you have infinite abilities will be valuable to you. Shifting your beliefs will benefit you and your body.

I told you about my gold medal gymnast vision, and I love doing cartwheels and handstands, and I love doing hand to hand acrobatics, but I don't feel inspired to try some of the more intense tricks that I never knew how to do. But I *believe* I can do them. I believe I can do them and I feel happy I can do them, but I don't actually do them until I feel super, super confident. I suppose the longer I believe it, the more I will feel compelled to try these tricks, but I never push myself, I just do what feels right in the moment.

Tell yourself that you can play that sport or do that activity you want to play. Tell yourself that you have boundless energy, that you are flexible, limber, supple. Imagine yourself doing the activities you want to do with grace and ease and energy. Imagine your body feeling the way you want it to feel.

And only take action when you feel one hundred percent confident that you can do it.

It's not really about the action, it's about feeling good about your abilities to do things.

Start affirming that "every day in every way, you are better, better and better."

Write out all the youthful improvements you find as you practice this new mental game and appreciate each improvement.

You will feel better and better, every day in every way!

Releasing the Cultural Hypnosis of Astrology

A lot of us have negative beliefs during certain times of astrological importance. These beliefs can hinder your body from thriving. They can block your energy and pleasure from being fully self-expressed.

I used to believe in astrology. I used to see negative things happening when mercury was in retrograde and on other astrologically scary times.

I remember one Vedic Astrologer who was supposed to be amazing at what he did told me a ton of negative things that were supposed to happen to me in the near future based on my vedic chart. I had met him when I believed in Astrology. Sure enough, I had taken his negative beliefs and put them on myself and I suffered, JUST LIKE HE SAID I WOULD.

That's called a 'nocebo.' A nocebo is a negative effect when you believe a negative diagnosis, prognosis or prediction. When you believe the nocebo, you get that negative result.

I feel so very, very thankful I now have total freedom from all negative programming from others by focusing on only what is relevant!

Then I started to live in unconditional love. As I did, I could feel all planets, stars, and the sky loving us. I could feel the moon loving us. I could feel all the world and the ground loving us all.

As I was walking in to teach a class on Living in Unconditional Love at the OneLoveFest one afternoon, I heard the people around me saying how everything was messed up because Mercury was in retrograde. I had felt everything flowing perfectly in my life, every day, in every way, for the last few years. I had had no idea Mercury was supposed to be affecting me negatively! I laughed out loud.

In that moment, I felt so thankful that I could feel that all planets, moons, stars, and other bodies in the sky love us all so deeply and unconditionally. They love us when they are moving in any and every direction. They love us no matter when we were born. We were all born under the luckiest, most fortunate stars! Once I felt that, I started to thrive more every day.

I realized that any negative experiences I had had from the stars or in any retrograde were my negative *beliefs* and *feelings* about the stars and planets and moons, or my negative thoughts about anything- not the actual stars and planets and moons. Now I feel total freedom and total consistent thriving no matter where any planet, star, or moon is or what direction it is going in! Every day is a lucky day for you and for me!

I also heard lots of people talking about how this time or that time was a very auspicious time when the veil between us and the cosmos was thinner… I feel so connected to all the cosmos all the time and have for years, that I realized that *every moment* is an auspicious time! There is no veil! We can connect with the entire cosmos at any time we desire. We are always fully connected to the entire loving cosmos, it's just a matter of opening to that awareness. It feels awesome to stay open to that all the time! Woooweee!

Practice 21. Releasing the Cultural Hypnosis of Astrology

Become aware of whatever it is you have believed about the planets, moons, stars, and other bodies in the sky and how they may affect you. If you believe it's a positive effect, then keep that belief. Allow yourself to release any thoughts or beliefs that do not lift you up and lighten you. As we learned in Practice 2, if it does not lift you up and lighten you, it cannot be the truth.

Allow yourself to perceive the pure love that all planets, moons, stars, and other bodies in the sky are all sending to you now and always. Allow yourself to know you are always fully connected to the Entire Universe. Allow yourself to know you were born under the luckiest stars. Allow yourself to see how all celestial bodies are all here for your total benefit *only*. They would only benefit you, they would never, ever hurt you. They *love you*.

Creating Your Own Hypnosis! What Not to Do

I heard a client talking about how something he was experiencing was really costing him a ton of money and was a pain in his neck.

What to Do:

In that moment I heard the phrase: "Pleasure in my neck."

Then I heard,

"Everything is benefiting me and prospering me. Everything is making me healthier and happier and richer. Everything is bringing me pleasure to my whole body. Everything is a pleasure to my neck!"

I shared this with him and after we laughed, we put it deep into his subconscious that this situation and all situations, circumstances, people, and things were making him richer, happier, healthier, and full of more pleasure.

He told me that this whole situation turned around within the next few days and that he was now much more conscious of what he said and that he loved programming himself to see everything as a benefit. He said he felt more energy, more abundance, and more health since that session.

I feel so thankful to all my wonderful clients.

Practice 22: Create Your Own Hypnotic Suggestions

You can program yourself to believe anything you want! You have been doing it unconsciously all your life. Now you can do it consciously in a way that benefits your amazing body.

Think about the kinds of things you want to believe. Get as deeply relaxed as you can. Then repeat your own hypnotic suggestions that lift you up and lighten you. You can repeat them silently or out loud, whatever feels best. Practice them consistently, right before you fall asleep, or right when you wake up, and any time, especially when you are deeply relaxed. Repeat them until these new thoughts become yours

– until it's a natural thought that you have for yourself with no effort. Practice them until it becomes automatic.

The more you become aware of the things you are hearing in the news, in your family, your work, your school, wherever you go, and the more you discern which things are lifting you up and lightening you, and the more you are letting go of the things that are not lifting you up and lightening you, the better you will feel, emotionally at first, then physically as well.

Identifying the false beliefs that are propagated by some media and unsuspecting people and then deliberately choosing which thoughts you want to release or practice feels so liberating and so empowering.

I feel so much love for you and you do not need to succumb to the negative experiences that our culture sometimes programs into us.

Create your own cultural hypnosis for yourself and watch your body and your life *thrive*!

This poem I wrote after realizing that the stars and planets loved us:

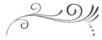

Do You Know?
The sky just whispered into my ear
a secret
that I vowed not to share –
but I cannot stop myself!
This is what the sky told me:
"Do you know
that I admire
You
with all my heart?
That the earth,
as you step upon it
reveres
You

and appreciates your divine connection with it?
Do you know
that the flowers are exuding their fragrance
to remind
You
how much they celebrate
You?
Do you know
that the air
as it flows into
You
is in rapturous adoration of
You
and of every cell of your being?
That the water
that washes your body
is in ecstatic bliss
at the chance of getting to have such intimate contact with
You?
Do you know
that all the food that this beautiful planet has provided for
You
is in such absolute admiration of
You
and is so thrilled to be consumed by
You
and to ravish your body
from the inside
with its perfect love?
Do you know that the sun is shining upon
You
saying to

You
with its warmth:
'You,
YOU,
You, my Precious One –
You
are the love of my life!
You
are the one I cherish with all of my heart!
You
are the one that I say,
'yes,
Yes, my love' –
to your every desire.'"
Now that I know this
There is nothing left to do but
be thankful.
By Karen Lorre

Chapter 8:

Pleasure is the Antidote to Pain

Pleasure is the antidote to pain. As you can see, every chapter before this has been focusing on finding new pleasurable thoughts, new ways to look at things in most every area of life.

Pleasure comes in many forms. There is physical pleasure, pleasure in eating healthy, nourishing, tasty foods, pleasure in a great conversation with someone you enjoy. There is pleasure in exercise, pleasure in being out in nature, pleasure in listening or playing or dancing to music. There is pleasure in meditation and pleasure in appreciating anything. There is pleasure in massage or other forms of touch. There is pleasure in singing, there is pleasure in much art, there is pleasure in animals and pets and children. There is intellectual pleasure, there is emotional pleasure, there is the pleasure of fragrance. Beauty is pleasurable. There is the pleasure of sexual and sensual sensations. There is pleasure in work that you love. There is the pleasure of ease and there is so much pleasure in anything that you enjoy.

I had been focusing on pleasure just because it feels soooo wonderful, and all the pleasure was in all the various forms written above. The more pleasure I felt, the less my body could experience pain. I was noticing how things that used to hurt me were not hurting me at all.

In fact, I had an accident where the tendons on the back of my hand got severed. I had a large gash, but I had no pain. I was planning on going bike riding that day, so I was just going to get a butterfly band aid. (I didn't know the tendons had been severed.) My neighbor came over and saw it and sent me to the ER. He said I needed stitches. I was so surprised. The ER docs told me that the tendons had been severed, but they could not fix it; I needed a specialist. The asked me how many pain pills I wanted. I didn't need any. They were amazed. After the surgeon fixed it, I still had no pain. I went to hand therapy and they asked me to rate my pain from one to ten. I said, "What pain?"

Yes, it took time to heal and I had to work to get the flexibility back in my hand but the whole process was super fun and I made some dear new friends and had wonderful experiences because of it. And having that experience made me really know that I could write this book to the depth of my being. I knew that what I had been practicing *REALLY WORKS!*

My body and brain had been so saturated in pleasure that even when this contrasting experience happened, I basically had no pain.

How does this happen?

My dear friend Norma Eckroate, had told me about two doctors whose workbook she was studying. Their names were Dr. Moskowitz and Dr. Golden. Norma had given me a link to their website and had let me look at the workbook, *Neuroplastic Transformation*, that Dr. Moskowitz and Dr. Golden wrote together. I went directly to the last tab of the workbook, which was entitled 'Pleasure.'

Moskowitz and Golden said, *"When pleasure rules there are responses that reverberate through pleasure areas, including the prefrontal cortex, anterior cingulate cortex, insular and amygdala, also part of the pain circuit. Releasing pleasure molecules counteracts release of pain molecules, making enjoyable experiences, happiness, love, hope and altruism such excellent pain relievers."*

They went on to say, *"Endorphins are neurotransmitters that are produced during exercise, pain, sexual activity, love and excitement.*

They are considered an important molecular component of the pleasure circuits in the brain. Endorphins are located in every part of the brain... Endorphins act as neurotransmitters attaching to opioid receptors which are located on nerve cells and astrocytes.... These important brain chemicals also regulate mood, motivation and reward systems in the brain. They are freely released during pleasurable experiences as well.

...The more activated the endorphin system, the greater pleasure we experience. Endorphins are released by the expectation of pleasure... Oxytocin is a molecule that exists on both sides of the Blood Brain Barrier, too large to cross between body and brain.... Recent studies have shown it to be important in pain, stress, mood stability, trust, pair bonding, parental behavior and love... Additionally it is a major stimulus for human sexual response in the peripheral body and brain.... It also appears to be involved in romantic love, romantic pair bonding and trust in brain pleasure circuits.... It plays a critical role as a social facilitator."[2]

I felt so excited when I read that.

Because we have neuroplasticity, when people focus on pain or even painful thoughts, for example, they actually grow their pain centers.

Some people grow their pain center so much that it's challenging for them to experience pleasure.

But I had intuitively done it in the opposite direction, by focusing so much on pleasurable emotions and pleasurable experiences that I had grown my pleasure centers; I had activated my endorphin system massively. I feel rewarded in every moment, even just washing the dishes! And I feel like I have an abundance of oxytocin, because when you love everyone and everything you feel bonded to it all, and oxytocin is all about bonding. Dr. Moskowitz and Dr. Golden's workbook confirmed and explained my experience.

They said that when you fund your pleasure centers by focusing on things that give you healthy nourishing pleasure (instead of using

---

2   Moskowitz, Michael H., and Marla DePolo Golden. *Neuroplastic Transformation Workbook.* 1st ed. Neuroplastic Partners, LLC, 2013.

things like drugs or alcohol or sugar or cigarettes that can harm you), as you fund your pleasure centers, they grow and grow and grow and they end up hijacking the pain centers so that they don't get activated much.

I realized that I had grown my pleasure centers so much that my pain centers are now just used as a basic communication:

"That flame is hot, stay back." "Pay attention to where you are walking so you walk around the coffee table." "Sit up straighter so your back is supported." Etc.

My trick for making sure all the pleasures I am doing are nourishing to me is that I make sure I feel my heart is soft and open, my brain is more receptive than active, and my body is relaxed, and I feel the connection to my Inner Divinity before I take any action. (More about that later.)

This is basically what this whole book has been about and is still about. Keep focusing on anything that gives you any form of pleasure, whether emotional, intellectual, physical, or any kind, and your body will not be able to experience pain the way it used to.

Case History

A beautiful client had a brain tumor that was quite painful, and he had tinnitus. The meds no longer worked to stop the pain, so he had been in agony. I coached him about funding his pleasure centers. After we worked together, I provided a recording that he could listen to that felt very soothing and pleasurable.

This is what he wrote me after our first session and listening to that recording I made:

"KAREN LORRE!!!!! AMAZING, LOVE, 'Funding the pleasure center,' I had NO idea... wow... okay, so, I started your meditation on the phone, put the top of my phone on my forehead and closed my eyes while I was

listening... the constant pain I'm always in decreased and the dreadful tinnitus, GONE! While you were talking... I gotta say... I actually felt better, this is a big deal for me now. Not thinking about this thing growing in my head was great, man, how cool is that. So, Karen Lorre... thank you so very much. You're not only beautiful on the outside, more importantly... you got it on the inside tenfold! Very cool I have it now to listen to when I'm feeling super bad or anytime. Okay, I've gone on long enough so, just have to say thank you thank you THANK YOU... Peace & Love Karen..."
Jason

I feel so very blessed to be able to work with so many wonderful clients and to see them thrive in new ways! I feel like the luckiest girl in the world!

Practice 23. Finding Pleasures You Can Do Easily

The more you find ways to feel pleasure, the better your body will feel.

Do Practice 1, Heartfullness Meditation. Focus on keeping your heart soft and open, feeling your mind receptive, your body relaxed, and a connection with the Source within you, and then take any actions that feel pleasurable.

Make a list of your favorite pleasures that are nourishing and healthy and make sure to do a few every day throughout your day. Each time you do a pleasurable action, or a pleasurable mental thought practice, appreciate yourself. Tell yourself you are benefitting your body and your whole life by feeling this pleasure. You are prospering yourself by feeling this pleasure. Do it often.

Some pleasure activities you can do while you are doing other things, like the pleasure of appreciation. Some pleasure activities take just a moment, like breathing in a wonderful essential oil or candle or fragrance for about a minute. Each time you take any pleasurable action you are funding the pleasure centers and therefore reducing your ability to experience pain unless it is the necessary pain of communicating something you need to adjust.

I believe that is what pain was originally meant to be for, a basic one-time communication that just guides us to what we want, not an incessant alarm that never goes off!

Case History:

I worked with a beautiful client, Jennifer, who wanted to learn to love more unconditionally. This is what she wrote:

> *"I asked for a meditation to help me to live more in love, more in my heart all the time ¬ and who better to ask than the Queen of Loving herself, Karen Lorre.*
>
> *Karen embodies true love and you can feel it in her buttery, delicious voice. Listening to my guided meditation is like going to the soul spa, like being wrapped in a velvety blanket of adoration. The words Karen chose resonate deeply with me, as the crystal bowl tones reverberate in my body. The words continue to resonate during the day, and with each listening new nuggets are revealed, new gems perceived.*
>
> *I've listened when I felt amazing and it took me higher; I've listened when I needed a tune up and the meditation re-aligned, re-calibrated, re-set my being. When I listen to my personalized guided meditation, I feel like I journey to the energetic essence of the experience of my most fulfilled, realized self, true and luminous self. Karen's voice guides me on an inner/outer*

journey of unfolding and enfolding layers of revelations and pulsations of pleasure. She tunes into the heart of my heart's desires and weaves them into the vision of the meditation."
Jennifer Mason

Blissipline

I have talked about a lot and it may feel overwhelming, contemplating all the things I have suggested. These were all done by me rather intuitively and they always felt fun. They were done over many months and years, so I encourage you to do the practices that feel the best and repeat them in a way that feels good for as long as you can – until you feel like it has become your second nature.

People often tell me that I have a lot of discipline to be as aligned as I am. I laugh. I do not use discipline to get things done. I never want to do anything out of obligation or force myself to do anything. I have found that counterproductive and I love you so much, I would never want you to do anything out of obligation nor to force yourself into anything.

Instead, I use what I call "Blissipline." Blissipline feels like pleasure. It feels effortless, it feels easy, I feel totally supported by the Universe, I feel fueled, and it feels absolutely like the Universe is doing the work as I do whatever action I am doing under the amazing magical powers of Blissipline. Blissipline feels like the Universe is my magic carpet ride and it's carrying me to take only inspired actions that feel like pure pleasure. This book is being written using Blissipline! I feel epic pleasure and pure love as I am writing this.

The way that I harness this Blissipline, and that I encourage you to do as well, is to use your brilliant mind to focus on all the things you love about something before you do it.

So, for example, to write this book, I would say something like this to myself:

"I love the feeling of flow, of the words downloaded into me. I feel so happy, writing from my heart that is full of love for you. I love feeling so delighted by what is coming through me as I discover it as it is being written. I feel blessed, it feels like I am taking dictation from my Inner Being. I love feeling attuned to you, Inner Being, so that I allow myself to perceive every subtle communication you are providing me."

I would say that or some version of that a few times, then I will feel compelled to do the action. The action will be inspired by my love for it.

Harnessing Blissipline can be used for doing any of the practices listed in this book. For example, if you want to make sure you do the practice of ascribing the qualities of Source to yourself, (Practice 11 – Chapter 6) you may say to yourself something like this:

"It feels wonderful to recognize and deepen my connection to who I really am. It feels amazing to write out all the qualities of Source and know they are mine even if I am still in the process of receiving them. It feels exciting to watch how my life is changing for the better as I become more and more of my Inner Divinity. I love how I feel more of my power as I ascribe my Source Energy qualities to myself...." And as you write your version of that out or say your version of that to yourself, you will feel so eager to start writing out all the wonderful qualities of Source Energy and ascribing them to you. That's the power of Blissipline.

I use it for every area of my life. Before I take any action, whether it is washing the dishes, or making dinner or exercising, working, seeing someone, or going to a party, I focus on what I love about that situation. I focus on all the good feelings I get from doing it. As I do this, my energy to do that thing increases. And then when I do whatever it is I am doing, I feel so supported, effortless, and in the flow as I do it.

I encourage you to do this on reading this book and doing the practices. The more you use Blissipline to do the practices the faster and more thoroughly your body will release all pain and fatigue and move easily into vibrant energy and chronic pleasure. And of course, do it on every area of your life! Never force yourself to do anything because you should do it or you need to do it or you have to do it. Use Blissipline to feel into how absolutely fun it will be to do it!

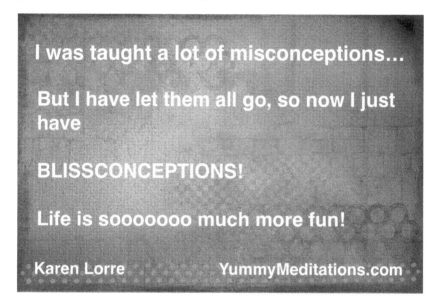

I was taught a lot of misconceptions...

But I have let them all go, so now I just have

BLISSCONCEPTIONS!

Life is sooooooo much more fun!

Karen Lorre   YummyMeditations.com

Practice 24. Harnessing the Power of Blissipline

What is the next thing you want to do? Or what is something you want to do but have been procrastinating? Or maybe pick something you will do in the future.

Write out or feel within yourself all the good feelings you will have as you do it.

Write out or feel within yourself the things you enjoy or love about doing that thing.

If you have never done it before, write out or feel within yourself the way you want to feel while doing it and after having done it as if you are feeling it already.

For example, if I was doing something new, let's say, talking to the UN, I may say to myself, "It feels amazing to be fully self-expressed. It feels so beautiful to speak from my heart so people can *feel* me. It feels wonderful to have total clarity on what I want to say. It feels so fun to express something never expressed before. It feels beautiful to see everyone's eyes light up as they listen and to feel their hearts open to this new truth...."

Write out your paragraph and read it to yourself a few times, or feel it and say it to yourself until you feel it is yours, you own it, it is natural for you. Say it to yourself before you are going to experience that action. If it's an action you do often, then memorize your paragraph and repeat it often.

Watch how every area of your life becomes easier and more productive as you employ the effortless, pleasurable magic of Blissipline. Watch how your body thrives in new ways, and so will your money and your relationships.... WOOOHOOOO YOU!

Relaxation

Relaxation is so important to pleasure! I took this strange but really fun fight class – not because I want to fight anyone, but because the class is all about relaxation, momentum, surface tension, and leverage.... All these things (except surface tension) I use emotionally, and they all enhance my life.

In my fun fight class, a big emphasis of the class is being totally relaxed and also aware of the other person and being aware of what direction their body is going. When you know that direction, you know what to do.

My teacher had me and a friend stand next to each other with our bodies tight, all our muscles engaged, and our eyes closed, and he told us to try to discern what movement he was doing. He put his hand on our shoulders. He made a movement.

Neither one of us could feel it at all.

Then he had us relax our bodies and he did the very same movement. It was subtle, but we could totally feel it and easily discern where he was and what direction his body was going. This meant that we knew what to do.

In that class, as I practiced staying physically relaxed, I found I could easily get any man who was much bigger, taller and stronger than me, onto the ground, effortlessly. It felt revelatory!

I love bringing deep relaxation into any situation where I want clarity and where I want to feel my inner guidance. I love how this class enhanced my already deep emotional relaxation into a deeper physical and emotional relaxation. I am so thankful for this amazing experience. The more relaxed I feel, the more attuned to pleasure I am. I relax as deeply as I can each day and that has enhanced my ability to feel epic pleasure from the smallest movements.

Practice 25. Relaxation throughout Your Day

Consciously scan your body for any areas that are already relaxed and appreciate them, and then look for any other areas that want to relax more. Breathe into those areas that want more relaxation and just gently encourage them to soften.

Good posture actually allows you to relax more because your body is stacked bone upon bone in an aligned way. The bones take the stress instead of your muscles.

Keep an awareness of how your hands are gripping or not, for example, while you drive. See if you can hold the steering wheel with relaxation, with a very light, aware touch.

Feel your shoulders dropping as you give yourself a body scan a few times every hour; keep your jaw soft. Breathe deeply into your pelvis.

The more relaxed you are, the more you will feel the subtle inspirations from the Source within you. The more relaxed you are, the more attuned to pleasure you will be. And the more relaxed you are consistently, the more you will shift your entire physiology.

We have what is called a Physiological Set Point. It's the normal state of our body's level of stress. The more you practice relaxation, the more your Physiological Set Point will lower and lower, so that you will be able to have less and less stress and your body will be able to hold more and more pleasure. The less stress you have, the better you are able to receive the impulses from the source within you.

Meditation feels like a wonderful practice to keep your body relaxed. I have been meditating two times a day (most days) for twenty-eight years at the time of this writing. My body knows how to relax deeply, so I get a great attunement to the subtle pleasures and inspirations from Source Energy.

Pleasure from Source

I felt so relaxed when I got this wonderful craniosacral massage. I loved the massage therapist's touch and the buzzing feeling I felt. Then, during our session, she started talking about something negative and I had no desire to hear that when I was in that deeply relaxed, receptive place.

When I got home, I was talking to my beautiful, brilliant friend, Shauna Mathis on the phone. I told her how much I loved the craniosacral massage and the deep relaxation.

I said, "God, I would love to experience that any time I want, with total silence and in my own home." As Shauna and I spoke more, I felt a gentle, subtle energy moving inside my brain.

I felt inspired to get off the phone, and I relaxed my body and closed my eyes and I could feel what I believe to be my Inner Being massaging the different areas of my brain – energetically.

As I felt this massage, this feeling of being caressed around and inside the structures of my brain caused my body to feel that same buzzing relaxation of the craniosacral massage. It felt like my Inner Being was massaging my lizard brain/ the brain stem/ the reptilian brain... Soothing it, loving it, renewing it, rewiring it, purifying it.

Every day, I was feeling this gentle, soothing massage in the brain stem and around it and as it was massaging me it felt like my whole brain stem was becoming a new structure in my brain. It felt amazing.

I felt like my Inner Being was cleansing my brain stem, removing all old patterns that were no longer needed. I felt a new innocence, a pure sweetness. I felt so loved.

My body was moving into the most quiet, tranquil experience I had ever had. Each time the brain stem was massaged, I felt my whole physiology drop into deeper restfulness. I felt like my instincts of fight or flight had disappeared. I now feel 'relax, or relax more' when something I don't want comes.

As this progressed, my Inner Being then massaged my corpus callosum – the bridge between the left and right hemispheres – so that I was always having full brain awareness, both hemispheres were being activated in a soothing rhythm. I can feel this gentle, soothing massage, while I write.

Now, my Inner Being massages me everywhere in my body and brain. It feels incredible and I can feel this massage when I am working or driving or doing *anything*. And because it is energy and not just physical, this massage can happen within or around any part of the body, this energy can go where no human touch can.

It feels a little too intimate to share all the places my Inner Being massages me, but you can try this out for yourself and find out what you like!

Practice 26. Receiving Internal Caresses

Lie down. Relax your whole body. It's best to do this after you already feel loved and nourished emotionally, so do the Heartfullness exercise if you want to feel more loved.

Ask your Inner Being to caress you anywhere you'd like. Feel your body relaxing deeper. Feel the tranquility that comes when you are totally focused on sensation.

(If you experiment with this enough, you will see why it's too intimate to share the specific places I get massaged with you!)

Allow yourself to feel this as if it was actual physical touch.

If you don't feel it right away, that's okay, just relax and *imagine* you feel it. Imagine you are being touched exactly as you like it, wherever you want. Feel this loving energy soothing you, pleasuring you, making you feel amazing!

...ENJOY!

The more you do this, the more your body will become attuned to pleasure. There are many more areas of the body that can be erotic than most people think. If you let your Inner Being massage you each night before you go to sleep, or whenever you desire it, you will find your response to normal touch becomes much more pleasurable.

Turn On

For me, I found the soothing touch of my Inner Being so erotic and such a turn on that I got addicted to it. I find that being turned on at least some of the day provides me so much pleasure. I often take time in the morning to either allow my Inner Being to massage me sexually or I will touch myself. I don't touch myself with the intention to climax, though I might, I simply touch myself or let my Inner Being touch me until I am fully aroused. Then I contract my pelvic muscles, drawing all that arousal into the rest of my body, and I go into my day with this extra passion and turn on and receptivity to pleasure. The more I do this, the more pleasure and energy my body feels. Even as I write, or drive or cook, or eat or work, etc, I can feel my Inner Being turning my body on. It feels rapturous to go through life like this!

Practice 27. Turn On

I can now experience this internal massage any time no matter what I am doing but to start off, it's good to be really quiet. Find a time you can be alone or with a partner.

Relax your body.

Allow yourself to get as aroused as slowly and gently as you can, in as relaxed a way as you desire. You can touch yourself or allow your partner or Inner Divinity to touch you. Allow yourself to be totally focused on the touch you are receiving so that you feel it fully, you are immersed in it, consumed by it. Allow yourself to be aroused and relaxed simultaneously. Keep relaxing your body the more turned on you feel.

When you feel aroused enough, so it feels really good, then either have an orgasm or contract your sexual muscles and pull that energy up your body. If you did not climax, you may want to use your hands to put pressure on your sex organs for a few moments to ground yourself, if you need that.

As you access that pleasure, you are telling your body that pleasure is important. Your body will start finding other ways that are perfect for you, to experience pleasure.

As a side note, after my Inner Being started massaging me regularly, that's when I simply lost my desire for sugar. It felt like life was so sweet that I had no need for sugar. I saw the sweetness in everyone and everything, and it felt like such a pleasure to see that sweetness so much that water tasted sweet, vegetables tasted sweet... Now everything I eat tastes so sweet. Pleasure is the antidote to pain, so the more pleasure you bring into your body, the better you will feel.

Transmuting Past Experiences into Jewels

When I was growing up, I went to a youth group at the invitation of a bunch of my friends. My family was not religious, I went for the fun of it. The minister who ran the youth group turned out to be a pedophile. He was mostly attracted to the young boys, but for some reason he also was attracted to me. I had harbored a resentment against him for most of my life. I felt that experience had hurt me in so many ways.

One morning I had been writing out all that I appreciated for about two hours. I had felt compelled to keep writing. I felt so high, so in love with the world. Then the thought of this man, Gary was his name, came to my mind. But instead of feeling that resentment, I saw the whole situation from the eyes of Source.

I could feel that if Gary had not told me he loved me while he was doing things to my body before I was old enough to desire them, I would not have had the strong strong desire to understand what real love really is and to learn to live in unconditional love like I do now. If Gary had not told me about God and how God loved me while Gary was being inappropriate, I would not have had such a massive desire to know what God really is (which is so much different than what Gary taught!), which had led me to having an intimate relationship with God (a.k.a. my Inner Being, my Source Energy, etc.) that has made my entire life magical.

And if Gary had not elicited or inspired the fear of men within me, I would not have had the burning desire to feel totally secure, totally relaxed, and totally confident with men, which is how I feel now and how I was feeling that day that I was full of appreciation, contemplating this experience of my youth.

In that moment, I felt the goodness of the situation. I realized he had inspired me to really have these incredible gifts and I was living with all those gifts consistently at that time and still now. I felt clear what love was and I felt and feel unconditional love ninety-nine point nine percent of the time. I felt totally clear what God is (as best as I can grasp it) and I felt that day and still feel a total communion with that incredibly loving power. And I felt and still feel this epic invincibility and confidence within me that Gary had actually inspired.

I also saw that at that time in my life, when I was in seventh grade, I had a lot of resistance to men and boys. I saw that my resistance, my defensiveness, attracted Gary to me. I had read lots of books at that age that were all against boys and men for some reason. So of course, I would attract that.

I fell to my knees in total appreciation at this realization. I saw that Gary was a divine gift to me; together we each had cooperated in that divine play. I felt the tears flow down my cheeks as I sobbed with the freedom of letting this whole pattern within me go. I realized there was no longer any need for me to forgive Gary or myself because I was seeing it all through love and I felt the perfection of him, of me and of the whole situation. Forgiveness was now moot. I did not need to forgive him – I only felt love and appreciation for him.

I felt like when you are working with clay and you remove the mold and the thing you are creating is there all pretty and clean… I felt like all sorts of resistance was falling away from me.

The next day, I got a Facebook message from Gary's wife. I had never been contacted by him or her and did not know they were even on Facebook. I had told no one of my new freedom, but they picked it up energetically. She asked if I would forgive Gary. She said Gary always loved me and that he was so sorry that I had been hurt. I read that message and just felt so much love and total awareness that I must have really shifted for her to reach out to me within less than twenty-four hours.

After that day, my physical energy increased massively. My sexual energy felt like it was flowing in a new, freer way. And more and more people were telling me I was radiant, glowing, lit up.

Practice 28. Transmute Past Experiences into Jewels

Get into a place of appreciation by doing any one of the processes that make you feel amazing, or your own practice.

When you feel saturated in thankfulness, simply ask to see the gifts in any experience that you want to feel better about. Ask this from your heart.

Ask this and listen not just with your ears, but with your whole being, and especially with your beautiful heart.

Allow yourself to *feel* the answers. Never try to get an answer, instead just allow yourself to receive the answer. It's a trick of letting go and being soft and relaxed when you ask, so that you can feel the new clarity with no effort.

Alternatively, if you don't yet feel able to receive the answers intuitively, look at the situation you want to transform and discern the things you were desiring at the moment that you were in that situation.

Know that all of your desires are immediately held vibrationally by your Inner Being. Your Inner Being had become that which you desire in that moment when that original contrast happened.

Write down the desires that you had had then. Look to see if you have already been living the fulfillment of your desires. If you have, give thanks and feel the appreciation for that experience. See how that experience made you who you are today in the most positive way.

If you have not yet fully allowed in all that you desire that was born from that contrast, that's totally okay. Relax, appreciate that now that you have identified the desire, you are automatically on the path for it to manifest. As Deepak always told me, "Inherent in every desire is the mechanics for its fulfillment." If you have a desire, it is destined to manifest. Know that all your desires that feel good are inspired by Source. All your desires are inevitable to manifest. You are right on track to manifest it – maybe a lot sooner than you think!

Appreciating Improvement

A lot of people put effort into making improvements in their lives. And they often get frustrated because the improvements are not coming as fast as they want. Do you ever feel impatient or frustrated about improvements? It's okay, you are right on track. And, there is an easier way.

This leads me to the wonderful practice of appreciating all the ways I have improved.

I found when I was trying to improve I would be using effort and nothing or very little would improve. Then when I gave up and just focused on the things that lifted me up and lightened me, things would magically improve. And when I started to appreciate improvements, the improvements kept growing. But again, I don't appreciate them to make them improve, I appreciate the improvements because it feels so fun to see how fast I am growing and evolving. I keep a note section in my phone for improvements.

Here is a list of some recent notes I made to myself about how I am improving:

- I feel so happy that I am understanding French so much better! And I feel so excited my pronunciation and accent are improving and my ability to express myself clearly is improving too! It feels more automatic! YAY!

- I feel absolutely over the moon that my hair is thicker and healthier, and it styles so easily now with no heat and still looks super cute! Thank you! I feel so delighted!

- I feel so thankful that I am becoming more flexible. YAY! That feels amazing!

- I feel thankful my eyesight keeps improving! I can read things that are so tiny or low contrast (white on light grey, etc.) and yet I see them clearly! YAY! I feel so excited!

- I feel so thankful that I am experiencing more and more pleasure and energy as I write this book. Writing feels so fun and flowing! I feel new passion and a whole new energy. YAY! Thank you!

- I feel thankful that my intuition is increasing so much. I have had so many intuitive synchronicities! That feels wonderful! Thank you!

- I feel thankful that my third eye is opening up so beautifully. I feel soooo clear! This feels luscious! Thank you!

- I feel happy that my communication with people is feeling more and more connected, from the heart and full of that bonded feeling of communion. I feel connected and delighted! Thank you!

If you notice, most of the improvements that I have appreciation for are not about my body, though some are. And in most of them I am not bringing in what it was like, I am simply noticing that it has gotten better or increased. This keeps my appreciation of these improvements pure.

A lot of people like to look back on what things were like before to see how far they have come and that is fine if you want to do that. But if you really want to keep improving, there is a bit of a paradox. Appreciating the current improvement fuels you for more improvements. However, when you bring into your mind what was not working, that can lower your current vibration. It's much better to simply focus on the aspects of improvements that you appreciate.

(And yes, I recognize that I have looked back throughout this book to share the way it was for me in the past before I applied these practices and understandings and I have practiced loving all that I experienced in the past so that it no longer hurts me to read or write it. I want you to know there was a path that really works. I want you to know that I understand where you may have been and that I feel confidence you can get to where you want physically, mentally and emotionally.)

And I use the word "appreciation" because it has a pure feeling. One definition of the word "appreciate" is "to rise in value." The more you appreciate anything, the more it rises in value – and so do you!

Even when I am not focusing on my body's improvements, my body is still benefiting by me appreciating the improvement in my French, let's say, or in my connected, bonded communication. Because I feel my heart opening even more as I appreciate my improvements, my open heart is causing my body to thrive in new ways.

You may have so many areas of improvement that you have not been aware of. It would feel awesome if you start to keep a running diary of *all* the ways in which you improve.

Practice 29. Appreciating Improvement

Get a note pad or use a page on your notes in your phone or computer.

Write out all the things you have seen improvements in. Describe your emotional feelings about the improvement (i.e.: I feel delighted that X has improved, or whatever you feel). As you write this, write it from your heart, feel your heart guide your awareness, and keep your body and mind relaxed and soft. Keep adding to this list every day that you see any improvements anywhere in your body or your life.

Watch as your beautiful body starts to feel more and more healthy, pleasured, energized. You will find yourself following inspirations that are specifically right for you.

Trust the inspirations you receive.

I can't tell you how many things I do that I was told *not* to do by so-called experts, but I feel inspired to do them and I watch my body thrive because of it.

For example, I was always told to be gentle with the skin under my eyes and around my eyes.

I have been gently exfoliating my face and body for a few years and recently I felt inspired to use a very coarse brush on my body. (It's actually a brush that is meant to clean other brushes – it has stiff long bristles.) The skin on my body *loved* it. Just a few strokes with this brush made the skin on my body turn red. That's a sign of good blood flow to the periphery. I felt inspired to try it on my face. The skin on my face *loved* it. I felt inspired to try it under my eyes. Not only does the area under my eyes *love* the way it feels, but that area started to look better. The skin tightened up and got lighter in color. Now the skin under my eyes and my facial skin look all the same color and texture. I am not saying you should do this, but I am saying that I listen to the inspirations I get, and I feel they all benefit me so much, even when it goes against what the experts or science says.

I do test them out in a very safe way first just to make sure. The first thing I do is make sure that the inspiration is a good-feeling inspiration. It's an inspiration that my open heart, full of love is perceiving. Then I may start slowly; for example, I started with that brush under my eyes for the first time with maybe three gentle strokes. Over the next few days, I slowly added a few more strokes and a bit more pressure under my eyes. Now I just treat the area under my eyes the same as the rest of my body and scrub with those tough bristles pretty hard. I feel delighted with how my skin is looking and feeling as I do this most days. If my skin is sensitive for some reason (which rarely happens), then I don't do it till my skin feels back to normal.

Practice 30. Trusting the Inspirations You Receive

The more you are relaxed, your heart is soft and open, and you feel the connection with your Inner Being, the more you will find yourself inspired to the things that are right for you. Trust your inspirations, your intuitions, *as long as they feel good*, and experiment in a slow safe way so you can discover any new secrets that really work for you and your precious body. We each have our own Divine Genius within us, and that Genius knows your body and knows what is right for you.

Each time you get an inspiration, and you follow it to some success, even a small success, write it down in the notes section of your phone or on in your computer or on a notepad. Make a running list that you can read over and over so that you can then re-activate your Inner Magic of following inspirations! Write out how they feel as you experienced them.

For example, I wanted some Lululemon yoga clothes but did not feel like going shopping. I did nothing. The next day my housekeeper came with a big bag and said, "Hey K, I got a big bag of clothes from another client. There may be a few things in here that fit you." I opened the bag and inside were tons of Lululemon yoga clothes with the tags still on, in my colors and my size. My inspiration had been to do nothing. I got everything I needed that day with *no effort*. That felt so easy and fun and I felt so catered to and pampered and so appreciative of my amazing housekeeper, Greyling Presley!

So write out each inspiration and how it makes you feel and read it any time you want to tap into your inspirations!

And listen to your body, listen to what it needs.

As I am writing this book, I feel my body's desire for movement, stretching, exercise every hour or two. I listen. Listen when your body wants you to eat a certain way or to drink more water or to do more meditation. Follow your inner wisdom.

This poem came to me while I was meditating:

As I was meditating, I felt my Inner Beloved say to me,
"Sweet One, I know you are seeking peace and quiet,
but I have other ideas for how you can use this precious
time..."
And I felt my body fill with energy that kissed me all over,
Penetrated me in the most surprising ways,
Coaxed out my most tender, sensitive parts,
Spread my heart open wider than I knew it could go,
Drenched me with hot, holy nectar
And caused ripples of luxurious waves
To flow up my spine
Infusing my mind with a bright, golden light.
Heck! Who wants peace and quiet when you can feel rav-
ished by God?
by Karen Lorre

Chapter 9:
Your Eternal Self

I had grown up believing that when people died, they were gone forever, that it was a terrible thing when someone died. I would get so depressed for months when someone I loved died. Then before I understood it intellectually, I started to have experiences that made me question that anyone or anything dies.

I have a wonderful client named Bethany. We worked together several times and had a sweet relationship. One day, I was half napping and I felt the energy of someone communicating with me. I got the feeling that it was Bethany's dad, who had died before I ever met her. I could hear him saying, "Tell Bethany she did the right thing. Tell her I am proud of what she did. She did the right thing. I am proud of her." I kept hearing him say that. I had no idea what that was about. I had not talked with Bethany for months. But I felt compelled to share it with her.

I tried to call Bethany, but I could not reach her. I decided to send her an email. I wrote,

"Dear Bethany, I got a message, I feel it was from your dad, but I don't know for sure. He kept saying, 'Tell Bethany she did the right thing. Tell her I am proud of what she did. She did the right thing. I am proud of her.'

Love, Karen"

Bethany called me so thankful. She had been out of the country doing a business deal, but she had not been sure if she had done it right. It was a deal with some business her father had left her. She had been crying in her hotel room, feeling so scared, wishing her dad was there so he could guide her, asking her dad for a sign – when my email came. She got her sign and she felt so relieved. She thanked me over and over. She later sent me a huge bouquet of flowers and a sweet card. I got off the phone wondering how that happened...

A few months later, I was driving in my car when I thought I heard a dog in the back seat. I pulled over to check, but there was no dog there. I got back in my seat to drive home and then before I pulled onto the street, I felt the energy of the dog that my ex-boyfriend and I had had together... Eli. Eli's energy was all over me; I could literally feel him licking my face and nuzzling me. Then I felt his energy saying, "Call Eric, you have to call Eric. You have to tell him he is going to get a dog and it's going to be me." My ex and I were recently separated, and I did *not* want to call him! I drove home and even as I was falling asleep, I kept feeling Eli licking my face and telling me the same thing. When I woke up in the morning, he was still there...

"Call Eric, tell him he is getting a dog and it is me." I could feel how elated Eli was... I finally called Eric.

"Hi Eric, it's Karen. Is this an okay time to interrupt?"

"Yes, I am just in the car."

"Okay... um. I got a message from Eli."

He didn't speak for a moment. Then...

"What'd he say?" He sounded wary.

"Well, he said that you were going to get a dog and it was going to be him."

Silence. I just waited. Then Eric said, "I am driving right now to San Diego to get a new dog." I could hear his heart touched as he said it.

I got off the phone, feeling amazed at the timing. I had no idea how it happened. These types of experiences kept happening. They happen so often it has now become normal.

However, this was happening when I was still sick, and the next energy I felt was my dear first real boyfriend, Johnny, who had been dead at that time for over ten years. I had mourned his death for a long time. In fact, my depressed reaction to Johnny's death had been one of the things that really made my body sicker.

This was a few months after I had been separated from my ex-husband. I missed my husband terribly. I had been feeling hopeless, suicidal. I had not known if I would ever be healthy again. I was unable to function at all. All my friends had stopped coming around and I felt so alone. I had not wanted to keep going.

As I was waking up one morning, I felt Johnny's loving energy. He was all around me. I could feel that he was communicating to me that life was worth living, that I would get better, that he would support me. I heard him start singing me a song that he had written to me when we were going out. (It's called 'I Feel the Magic,' and Belinda Carlyle sang it when she left the GoGos.) The lyrics he sang were: *"I feel the magic like I never felt before. I imagine that it's always been there. Like an angel looking after me. Angel baby give me more and more."* He had written it to me, as if I was his angel when we had been together…As I heard that, I felt a clear knowing that Johnny was now *my* angel.

I felt him guiding me with the foods I should eat. I felt him singing that song to me any time I started to go into a depression or get tired or negative. I felt him everywhere. He gave me hope when I needed it. He assured me life would be worth living again. He made me laugh when I had any resistance. I felt so very thankful to him.

At this point, I had not known yet about the Law of Attraction, but Johnny led me to it.

Johnny led me by my heart to my bookshelf and guided me to read everything I could about the Law of Attraction.

I did read that book, and everything began to make sense. I learned that there is no death, that everyone is simply returned to their true, loving nature and they drop all resistance, all false beliefs, all limitations, when they die. That made all the experiences I had been having finally make sense.

I still feel Johnny all around me, always singing to me, telling me funny things, making me laugh, pleasuring me.

When I would feel I needed a nap, I would lay on the couch and feel so upset that I was still tired, even after knowing so much about Law of Attraction. Then I heard Johnny and my Inner Being whispering in my ears while I was falling asleep on the couch one more time. "Karen, you are doing everything right. You are right on track. It's good for you to take a nap now. It's perfect. Just relax. Let your body relax. When you wake up, you will feel better and you can do something like writing out appreciation to give you more energy. Right now, you are doing everything right. There is nothing you need to do. There is no place you need to go. You are doing everything right. You have all the time in the world. Just relax, let your body relax…"

I heard this every time I got tired.

I realized I could also do this for myself. I stopped getting mad at myself for being tired and instead I would soothe myself like Johnny and my Inner Being soothed me. Johnny and my Inner Being and my narcolepsy taught me how to be kind and gentle with myself. Johnny and my Inner Being and my narcolepsy taught me to be kind and gentle with you too.

The more I did that, the more my energy increased, and I did not need many more naps. Now, if I take a nap, it's rare, maybe one or two naps a month, and I feel so blessed and happy to be able to do that. My naps feel amazing now.

After I learned the Law of Attraction, I was writing out my appreciation one night and when I got into bed, the room filled with so much love, it felt so thick, like I could cut the love with a knife. It felt undeniable. I felt that it was my dad, who had been dead for at least eleven years at that time. I felt my dad loving me way beyond any depth of love I had ever known. I felt him telling me he was proud of me. I felt huge sobbing tears of so much resistance and sadness leaving my body. I felt my dad so clearly.

And now I understood it. Of course he was there, of course he was pure love. Now, because of Abraham - Hicks, (Thank you!) it all made sense. My dad gave me so much love and so much affirmation. It felt like he was re-writing our history together. I could see my past with him in a totally new way. It felt like all that I could see were the times when we were laughing, playing frisbee, playing catch with the football, building the tree house together, building the playhouse together, doing acrobatics together, having fun. He shifted all the childhood memories I had so I could only focus on the happy, joyful, connected ones.

This shifted my relationship with my mom, my brother, and all my relatives. I felt a new love for them all. Somehow my dad shifted my whole memory of my mom too, so I could only see the ways she had been so fun, so wise, so loving and thoughtful and playful and sweet. All the fun times were highlighted. I couldn't even remember any negative times. This made my love for my mom increase.

My dad has inspired me to love my mom and my brother and his family in a whole new, deeper way than I had. He inspired me to ask my mom's friends and our family and the friends of my brother and me who love my mom to each write a letter to her about what they appreciate about her and send it to me. I had it printed into a hardcover book with all the pictures of each person with their letters of appreciation. It makes me cry to read that book, it is so full of love for my mom. I have always adored my mom, but my admiration and my appreciation for her really increased as I did that project. My dad inspired me to do that book for my mom. He knew it would increase the love she receives from me and from each person who wrote their appreciation in the book.

My mom said she reads the book every day and that she loves it. That makes me feel so happy.

And now, my dad, Johnny, and a host of other non-physicals are with me all the time.

There is no death. The first law of thermodynamics says that energy can neither be created nor destroyed; energy can only be transferred or changed from one form to another.

When anyone, or any animal or any plant 'dies,' who they really are is now transformed into a new nonphysical form. A form that is free of resistance. A form that is pure love, joy, bliss, wisdom, health, well-being, abundance, freedom, and everything that Source Energy is. This is what I had been feeling before I understood it.

Once I really experienced this knowing that no one dies, that their energy is in pure bliss and love, I got so much more energy and my body felt soooo much better. And the daily moment-to-moment contact I have with those 'non-fizzies' – as I like to call them – feels rapturous. Anytime I have a desire, I feel some non-fizzy here loving me and guiding me to it.

I live in a house on top of a mountain on a private road with no other house within a football field around me. Nature is all around me. People often come here and ask if I am afraid when I am here alone. I laugh. I don't tell them this, but *I am never alone*! The nonfizzies keep me so safe and secure and happy that I always feel completely connected and safe.

Practice 31. Connecting to Non-Physical Energy.

Do Practice 1, Heartfullness Meditation, for opening your heart. Allow your mind to relax and relax your body.

Bring your attention to your heart and ask to feel a connection with any person, animal or plant, or object that you want to connect with. Just relax and allow yourself to receive.

When you feel that energy, first just allow yourself to experience the depth of love, the total adoration that that non-physical energy has for you.

When you are ready, simply ask anything and then relax and allow the answer to come in. *Don't TRY* to get an answer, just allow the answers in.

This may take some practice to trust yourself that you are receiving accurately. One way to know is that if the communication you receive lifts you up and lightens you, then it is the truth. If it does not, then it is your own thoughts. These non-fizzies are always here to lift us up and lighten us. They are here to play! They are here to love us completely!

Keep practicing this until you find your resonance. You must be in the same frequency as the non-fizzy with whom you wish to connect. Which is why you would need to be in pure bliss, love, happiness, security, freedom, and fun to feel them. Once you get practiced at this, your life will feel even more magical and fun! The non-fizzies can make every area of your life incredible. They LOVE you and are here to support you.

The Truth About the Imposter Syndrome

Case History

I was coaching a brilliant and beautiful college-aged girl who was expressing that she felt she was an imposter. She felt insecure, like she didn't believe she was worthy of all the good things that were happening. She did not feel she had anything to contribute. She felt afraid to speak up.

I gave her a big hug over Skype. I felt so much love for her. I realized that she was accurate, she was being an imposter to who she really was. I felt so much love for her. I coached her on connecting with the Source within her and with ascribing to herself all the qualities that her Source Energy had. As she put this into daily practice, she started to glow. Her posture improved. Her energy increased. Her skin cleared up. Her confidence grew. She started to manifest all the things she was wanting. She became outspoken. She became her *real* self.

Imposter syndrome is when you forget the magnificent majesty and glory of who you really are.

The more you recognize that you are a divine being, that you are never alone, that you are always supported and loved, the more you recognize that there is no death, the more you will feel that vibrant energy within you. You will have that ability to be light and playful and fun. Your body will thrive in new ways.

You are never alone. In everything you do, there is both your Source Energy and all the non-fizzies who adore you. They love resourcing you, pleasing you, delighting you, clarifying you, inspiring you, prospering you (and so much more!) Be open to all the inspirations that are coming from your Inner Being and from all the non-fizzies that adore you. Keep your body relaxed, your heart open, your mind receptive and you will feel yourself being danced through your life. The ecstasy of who you really are is beyond comprehension.

Practice 32. Reaffirm Your Eternal Amazing Self

If you ever feel any sense of wanting to feel better about yourself, then simply go back to Practice 11, Bypass My Own Personality to See the Best in Me, and ascribe to yourself every wonderful quality that the Source within you has. I suggest you write it out daily until you feel saturated in your divinity, until you feel so sure of who you are, that it feels impossible to ever doubt yourself in any way. Write it out and affirm it to yourself so often that you feel unstoppable – *you are.*

Access Your Unconditionally Adorable Nature

I was driving and I was feeling a bit of resistance – negative emotion because of another driver. Or at least I was blaming my resistance on him. Now I know that my resistance is *my* responsibility, no one else's.

When I felt my resistance that day, I prayed to feel better. In that moment, I felt all the love in the Universe flowing into me. I realized my Inner Being was amplifying my ability to perceive the love my Inner Being had for me. I felt a bit surprised that I could feel this so clearly when I had just been having negative emotions, and I asked my Inner Being what was going on.

My Inner Being just poured more love into me, and then I understood that my prayer to feel better had worked immediately and it had caused me to release all the negative emotion so I could feel the pure love I was receiving. Then I got that I was loved so unconditionally, even with resistance. I felt the Universe telling me that I was so cute and adorable with my resistance. I felt my body relax even deeper, then I felt this knowing:

"It's true, you are loved unconditionally, even when you are in resistance, so you can relax, and know you are loved. Then when you have any negative emotions you can know that you are truly adorable, truly cute with that negative emotion. And everyone else is loved and adorable when they have resistance. This will bring you back into alignment."

I started crying with the recognition of how very unconditionally loving this world is. I felt so thankful, so very, very loved. And since then, whenever I feel any resistance, I just love myself and know I am totally cute and adorable while I am in it. That makes all my resistance dissipate so quickly. And I apply that to you and to everyone as well. If anyone is in resistance, I relax and know how absolutely adorable you are, or they are, and I flow my love to you, and to them.

Practice 33: Discover Your Unconditionally Adorable Nature

Know that you are loved, that nothing you can do can ever stop you from being loved. Even when you feel bad, you are being loved, you are adored, you are cherished and respected and valued, no matter what you feel. Next time you have any resistance, tell yourself, "I am so adorable when I feel like this." And enjoy that there is nothing that can ever stop you from being adorable and adored by the Entire Universe.

Invincible You:

As I meditated one morning, I felt my infinite nature in a new way. I realized I was much, much bigger than my precious body, I felt bigger than all of creation. As I felt this, my energy merged with all that is. I felt the complete tranquil silence and freedom of my being. I could feel that I am invincible. I felt a new wholeness within me. I feel so confident. I feel unstoppable. The more I felt that, the more that my whole body was vibrating in pleasure and vivaciousness. I realized that all of creation was only a speck in the magnificence of who we really are. And I felt this truth for everyone as well.

Because you are an infinite eternal being, your energy is bigger than all of creation. Creation is finite. You are infinite. This means that who you really are is more powerful than anything that is happening on this earth. Who you really are is more powerful than anything that is happening in your amazing body. You are Source Incarnate. You are that which created all that exists. You are unstoppable. You are invincible.

Practice 34. Experience Your Invincible Nature

Do Practice 1, Heartfullness Meditation, and open your heart, relax your mind so it's receptive, and relax your body. Make sure you are feeling loved and loving.

Now ask your Inner Being to let you experience your infinite, eternal, invincible nature. Allow your body and your mind to relax deeply, to feel as if they are dissolving as you expand out in every direction. Recognize that all of creation, all of the cosmos is only a tiny speck in the magnificence of your being. Realize that you are bigger, more powerful than anything.

Enjoy and savor this feeling.

The more you tap into your invincible nature, the more you will feel soooooo much more control of your health and your well-being. Your body is a reflection of your thoughts and as you feel that invincible nature more and more, your body will feel its own invincible nature. You will feel stronger, healthier, more pleasure, and more energy. It feels ecstatic to rest in your invincible nature. And knowing that you are so much bigger than any contrast or experience or condition that is happening can unlock so much more energy for you. You are an infinite, eternal being. You truly are unstoppable. You truly are invincible.

This is a poem I wrote after feeling that expansion the first time:

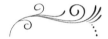

I feel held in the heart of God
Ensconced in rich, warm harmonies
That make my own heart
Sing
I feel, from this wondrous womb-like place
That there are no questions
I feel completely accepted exactly as I am
I feel completely loved exactly as I am
I feel merged with this Divine Heart
Like when I am in the ocean,
And the water feels the same temperature
As my body
And the air feels the same temperature too,
And I cannot tell where I end
Or where the ocean or the air
Begins...
I feel dissolved into the soft, warm waves
My mind has opened into pure silence
There is nothing I have to do
There is nowhere I have to go

I have always been perfect and evolving
Everyone has always been perfect and evolving.
Outrageous joy
Blooms inside me like the morning sun
I feel my invincible nature...
I am pure Bliss
I feel your invincible nature.
You are pure bliss
By Karen Lorre

Chapter 10:

Letting the Universe Do the Work

A   s you can see, so much of this book is all about your emotional experience and how that affects your body. Since I have been living in pure love, I have been inspired to so many amazing things that make my body and me feel even happier. I will share all my fun things in another chapter, but for now, I want to encourage you again to put these practices into action. The happier and more love-filled you feel, the more the things that are specifically right for *you* will come into your life. And in my experience, I did all these practices many, many times for years, but now I don't have to do much at all to feel the deep infinite connection with all that I am and to receive all that I want. I now rest in my pure, blissful Beingness.

As you do these practices, know that you are creating new momentum, which will help you, and that your brain is now going to be helping you more and more as well. These amazing feelings will feel better and better each time you practice them and the more you do them, they can become automatic.

Intuition

I had found that I was pursuing pleasure intuitively. I felt compelled to find things that gave me emotional pleasure, physical pleasure and gustatory pleasure, musical pleasure, conversational pleasure, breathing pleasure, massage pleasure, increased sensual and sexual pleasure, exercise pleasure, connection pleasure... I had literally felt compelled to make everything I did be as pleasurable as I could.

I had no idea why I had been so compelled to find pleasure in every way, until I was actually living in Chronic Pleasure, and then read some of Dr. Moskowitz's and Dr. Golden's workbook, *Neuroplastic Transformation*.

They said that pleasure blocks pain. Pleasure decreases inflammation, pleasure enhances the neurotransmitters that cause the feeling of being more bonded with people, to feel more trust, to feel more easily connected with people.

I had noticed that the more pleasure I had, the more all of my relationships thrived, the more bonded I felt with people, the more I felt at home everywhere I went. I love following my intuition and then finding out why I had felt so compelled to do something later.

I had intuitively had the thought:

"Everything is giving me more pleasure and more energy. Everything is a blessing for me."

My body became more and more sensitive to pleasure as I affirmed that. I felt giddy with pleasure more and more.

Then I read Dr. Moskowitz and Dr. Golden's book, *Neuroplastic Transformation* (neuroplastix.com), which says, *"Thus both pain and pleasure are not actually feelings, but are values placed upon sensation mingled with emotions and thoughts...' We are capable of producing pleasure and all efforts to do so should be directed at doing so.'"*[3]

This confirmed my intuitive desire to see that everything is giving more pleasure and more energy. Pleasure and pain are not exactly feelings, they are instead my interpretation, my opinion of whatever sensation I am experiencing. You can literally decide to perceive everything as a pleasure and the more you practice that belief, the more your body will respond with pleasure to every sensation you experience.

---

3   Moskowitz, Michael H., and Marla DePolo Golden. *Neuroplastic Transformation Workbook*. 1st ed. Neuroplastic Partners, LLC, 2013.

That's what I had done long before I read their workbook, but I felt so happy understanding why I had been compelled to find everything pleasurable after I read their workbook. (I am a bit of a science nerd, so I love this stuff!)

But here's the trick with intuition. If your heart is wide open, if it's filled with love, if you feel happy and blissful, and if the guidance feels good, then your heart will perceive the guidance accurately.

If your heart is closed and you feel an intuitive hit that does not feel good, or feels like concern or any negative emotion, I would suggest you wait, wait until you are able to open your heart, wait till you feel filled up with love, then ask again for the intuitive wisdom and see what you get.

When the heart is open and your intuition feels good, it will be more accurate. When your heart is closed, don't listen to your intuition because a closed heart will misinterpret the wisdom that is flowing in.

Our Inner Beings don't guide us with negative emotions, except to say, "Hey, you are feeling negative emotion, which means that you are out of alignment and need to get back into alignment. You are still lovable, you are still adored, but until you feel better, you are out of alignment."

When you get an intuitive feeling, it will be a positive feeling or a 'relax and do nothing' feeling.

For example, one time a friend and I were driving on a freeway in two separate cars. We had a plan to take another freeway in order to get to this event we were attending.

As I drove, I could feel my heart overflowing with love. Suddenly, I felt my body compelled to drive me toward the next exit, a few exits before the second freeway. I had no idea why I was going that way, but I felt full of love, so I decided to trust it and go with it. I exited off the freeway and was driving on city streets to get to the event when my cell phone rang.

My friend on the other end sounded confused. "Hey, the freeway we were going to take is closed... how do I get to that event from here?" she said.

At that moment, I realized why I had felt compelled to get off the freeway. I did not get warned that the freeway was closed; instead, I felt an overwhelming impulse to exit the freeway early. I gave my friend the directions and I got to the event on time and was able to save seats when she finally arrived.

That's what I mean about having intuitions that feel good. Intuitions must lift you up and lighten you, they must feel good and relevant for you to know they are accurate. Your intuition may not feel logical, but if it feels good, it's leading you to the most logical conclusion. The more your heart is soft, open, full of love and receptive, the more your brain is quiet, and your body is relaxed, the more your intuitive heart will guide you to what is right for you.

Be open to this intuitive guidance – again, as long as you feel good and the guidance feels good. It may not always make sense, it may go against what you have been taught; as long as it feels wonderful, trust it.

Practice 35. Developing Intuition

Do Practice 1, Heartfullness Meditation, until your heart feels soft, open, and relaxed. Then keep a gentle awareness on your heart as you go about your day. When you feel an intuitive hit, write it down and write down how you feel. If you feel ecstatic, if you feel happy, and especially if you feel compelled in a joyful way, then follow that intuitive impulse *at that moment.*

If you don't feel fabulous, make a note of it and just go do the next inspired thing that will make you feel better emotionally. As you keep your heart more soft, gentle, and open, you will find your intuition more and more clearly. For me, it often feels like my body is being pushed or pulled energetically. Sometimes I hear a voice that guides me. Sometimes I feel the emotions that guide me. Sometimes my head is gently turned in such a way to see something that is 'lit up' for me and I feel compelled to go in that direction.

Any time you have an intuition that you follow that leads you to something you want, make a note of it. I have a notes section in my phone and computer that is just called 'Intuition.' Each time you get an intuition that is accurate or leads you to what you want, write it in that note section or in a notebook and appreciate it. Everything you appreciate grows in value, so the more you appreciate it each time, the more you will be able to discern the intuitions that are true guidance and the intuitions that are inaccurate. That discernment will increase every time you write down the intuitions that have led you to what you want and appreciate them. The intuition that is inaccurate will simply fall away with practice.

Your Every Thought Is a Prayer for More of That

I had a client who was talking about prayer. She said she spent time every morning praying for what she wanted. Right after she said that she started to complain about something that was not working in her life. She was trying to figure out what she was doing wrong.

As she was talking, I felt such gentle compassion and clarity. I could see that she was counteracting what she prayed for with her awareness of what was not working and with her trying to figure out what was going wrong.

One key thing that had really helped me was when I realized that my every thought, emotion, and action was a prayer for more of whatever I was thinking, feeling, or doing.

I felt excited when I had seen how I had mixed prayers all the time… sometimes thinking of what I wanted and sometimes thinking of what I did not want. Sometimes taking actions that felt good and sometimes not. It felt so clear why I had been only getting some of the things I wanted, but not all of the things I wanted.

I had felt excited because once I saw how I was not always focused on what I wanted, I felt clear that it could shift. I felt devoted to shifting it so that I was as close to one hundred percent pure in each moment, focused just on what I wanted.

As my client and I talked, and I shared with her that every thought, emotion, and action is a prayer, even when you are driving or working or reading the news, or listening to the lyrics of a song, she had one of those beautiful 'aha' moments – her eyes lit up and this beautiful smile blossomed on her face. She looked ten years younger almost immediately and so very beautiful.

We talked about asking questions that feel really good to ask instead of trying to figure out what was going wrong.

I suggested she ask questions like:

- How good can I feel?
- How much fun would it be when X manifests?
- How fun and easy can life be?
- How much pleasure can I feel?
- How healthy can I be?
- How successful can I be?'

You don't even have to answer any of the questions…

Just asking those fun types of questions causes you to tune to the energy of the answers, which causes you to feel better emotionally, which causes you to feel better physically! It's another luscious cycle!

My client got so excited and she began to really feel her power as she practiced knowing every thought is a prayer and making sure she was praying for what she wanted.

Every thought, emotion, and action is a prayer. That means that 24/7 the Universe is feeling your energy. There is no time when you are not praying.

Practice 36. Your Every Thought Is Your Prayer

Make a list of thoughts you really like, write them down in your phone or computer or on a piece of paper, and keep a running list that you can read over whenever you need to refocus your mind. If you see a thought that really makes you feel good, add it to your list and keep adding it so you can just read it over and over and entrain yourself into a new truth. Each time you read your list, you are bringing all of that to you – as long as you read it just because it feels good, and not to bring all you desire to you! Giggle!

Practice 37. Asking Questions that Feel Good

As you drive or as you are doing something like cooking or walking, silently or out loud, ask yourself questions that feel really good to ask.

For example:

- How happy can I be?
- How much pleasure can I experience?
- How intuitive can I be?
- How rich can I be?
- How much fun can I have?
- What magic is here for me today?

Just ask yourself anything that lifts you up and lightens you. Ask yourself relevant questions! Have fun with this. All these practices are meant to be done with playfulness, lightness, and fun!

Heartfullness vs. Mindfulness.

Being aware that every thought, emotion, and action is a prayer requires a total awareness of what is happening within your mind, body, and emotions. It requires that you be very, very present to yourself. Minding all your thoughts can feel like a challenge.

The very first practice I gave you, the Heartfullness Meditation – about opening your heart – feels so valuable to me because it bypasses my need to monitor my thoughts, which feels too cumbersome.

Keeping my attention gently on my heart throughout my day and making sure it feels soft, open, receptive and full, keeps my mind tranquil and receptive and my body relaxed. That's why I practice and teach Heartfullness instead of Mindfulness.

Keeping your heart open, soft, and full will keep your mind relaxed and receptive to the genius of your Inner Being, so that you will be more in the flow. You will have the experience of just BEING. It will also make your alignment feel more physical, it will get that feeling of love inside your body, instead of it being an intellectual thing.

As we talked about before, the heart is intuitive, it knows things before the brain can see it, hear it, taste it, touch it, or feel it. That's really a huge reason why I practice Heartfullness, plus it feels so beautiful to have my heart feeling so full of love as I go about everything I do. It feels wonderful to write from my heart, to speak from my heart and to listen from my beautiful, sacred, loving heart.

I encourage you to keep your attention – at least in part – on your amazing, intuitive heart, so that you can follow the gentle inspirations that will guide you to all that is right for you. When your attention is on your heart, you may feel that warmth in the center or the left of your chest. You may feel the beat of your heart, you may feel the relaxation there in the center left of your chest.

For me, it feels like my heart is shining out in every direction, shining like the sun.

If it's hard to keep your attention there, practice putting your hand on your heart and discerning the gentle rhythmic beat of your heart, then making sure your heart feels soft, relaxed, open.

For me, I can feel any tension in my heart/ chest area so quickly because I have my attention on my heart so much now. It feels so easy to be aware if I have tension and then to let it go by breathing into my beautiful heart with soft, gentle kindness. I can let go of tension so quickly because I feel it at the moment it occurs, and I always let it go as soon as I am aware of it.

Your body is listening to everything you say and think and feel and do, and it is responding to it all the time. Your body has the capacity to transform so very quickly.

My Amazing Client's Story

I was working with a client who had comedonal acne and she wanted it to clear up. So we did some coaching where she learned to focus in a more heartfull, pure way, and I created a meditation for her on beauty, which is what she was really wanting for her skin. I suggested she listen to it over and over, which would then train her brain and body into what she wanted.

Here's what she said:

> *"I never met Karen Lorre before contacting her for a personal meditation session. What follows is my real-life experience after doing a [coaching and] meditation with her on beauty!*
>
> *I've had comedonal acne since age twelve and I tried every physical remedy and went to many dermatologists and nothing budged. After hearing about Law of Attraction I figured I had it for an emotional reason but could never manage to cure it.*
>
> *The few following days from my guided meditation and [session] with Karen on beauty, for the first time it's [Comedonal acne] literally disappearing from my face. After only two days it's about fifty percent better. When I looked in the mirror, I couldn't believe it, it's just falling away! I honestly did not expect such a fast result.*
>
> *Furthermore, my face just looks so different already to me and people are telling me I look beautiful. I look radiant, the structure of my face is more attractive and symmetrical. I have the look of a cute*

angel-like version of myself that I've always longed for
and also the redness on my face is gone!! Really every-
thing is so malleable, and age doesn't matter, Karen
has taught me that in a powerful way! My skin kept
getting smoother and better as I listened to the med-
itation. It's in a state now that I like it. I am so glad I
found her and would recommend her meditations and
guidance to anyone!!"
    Ellen Hutchersen

Practice 38. Heartfull Awareness Throughout Your Day

Since your every thought is your prayer, you want to be aware of your thoughts, but also be easy about it. The more you keep your gentle awareness on your intuitive brilliant heart, the easier it will be. Just having your awareness there and making sure your heart feels full of love, wide open, and shining love like the sun, will keep your thoughts naturally in alignment with what you want. If you keep attention on your heart you will feel if your heart starts to get tension or to close, and you will know to gently breathe softness into it, breathe kindness and warmth until you feel your heart again soft and full of love and open. In this way you will be guided to more aligned thoughts and negative patterns will begin to disappear.

Visioning

I remember my high school gymnastics coach had taught me to visualize whatever I wanted to do in gymnastics so that I would be able to do it. The night before a workout or competition, I would lie in my bed trying to picture what I wanted. I noticed that sometimes my visualizations really made the next day's tricks work better and some days they didn't. I wondered why it worked or not.

As I learned about the Law of Attraction, I realized why the visualizations I had tried throughout my life worked only some of the time and not always. When I discovered the secret, I felt amazed at how simple it was to shift it so that everything I visualize comes to pass in its own way and its own time.

Here's what works:

Through my acting career, I learned something called Sense Memory. It's where you can imagine having, for example, a lemon in your hand, and you can feel the weight of it, the coolness, the texture of its peel, you can smell it, see it, you experience it in its totality. Then imagine cutting it in half and in quarters. Smell one of the quarters. Then take a bite of it. Suck on that quarter of the lemon like it's an orange... do you feel your mouth already getting more saliva? That's how fun it is to visualize and how responsive your body is.

That's the technique I use to envision what I want in my life, but with a catch!

I must feel totally in a state of love before I start to envision. Then, I create a vision, I envision it in every modality that I can, so I hear it, see it, smell it, taste it, touch it, feel it... I allow it to feel real...

Then I practice the visualization until it feels so real and easy that it feels like the truth.

But here's the trick: *I don't visualize anything to make anything happen. If I am trying to make something happen with a vision, then I am really telling the Universe that I don't like the way something is, which will give me more what I don't want. What we resist, persists.*

And if I think it should manifest at a certain time, then I am always 'checking the temperature of the dish' too often and disrupting the cooking... so I take time out of the equation and I make sure that I do the vision simply for the joy and pleasure of doing it in this moment.

The other aspect to envisioning something is that I experience the vision the way I want it, while I am feeling full of love and happiness at the same time. If I feel any negative emotion, then that is a sign that

I need to get back into alignment and after I am back in alignment, I envision what I want when I am feeling good.

I can envision any result I want, but I never envision to make anything happen.

I envision something in the future, in order to feel good now. I envision something new from the past, in order to feel good now.

Feeling good now is the only reason to envision (or to do) anything.

But then because you feel good, the essence of that thing will come to you.

It may not be the exact person, or place or job, etc. but it will be something that has the same emotional frequency that you do. Always start by being in a state of love, and only what you love can come to you.

Never visualize to make anything happen. Visualize to feel even better now.

Let it unfold as it unfolds. Do not check or monitor or keep score if it is unfolding or not. Trust that it is unfolding in the perfect way at the perfect time.

That's the secret to visualizing.

There's one more secret to visualizing that can happen:

It's when you are not visualizing but you are in alignment and you *receive* a vision of something that's coming to you.

When you have that experience, that's when you record every nuance of that vision and then keep envisioning it when you feel good. That's when your Inner Being is really giving you knowledge of what is coming. It feels amazing how perfectly the Universe sends the info of what is coming. Each time it happens, I feel blown away by the perfection and feeling of being psychic. I have received visions of people and houses and experiences I am going to have before I have them so that when I arrive and I see, for example, that the house is *exactly the same house that came to me in my meditation*, so that I knew how many bedrooms and fireplaces and what kind of kitchen it had when I was still in my car, before I had ever entered the house. It makes me take note and realize that this is something that is here for me.

A Fun Example of How Visioning Affects the Body

When I was working as an actress on the soap opera *One Life to Live* as Tina Lord Roberts, I played pregnant at one time. I wore an ever-increasing sized pillow stuffed under a leotard under my clothes for many months Because it was under my clothes, it was too hard to remove and then put back on when I went outside the studio to lunch. So I often went out to lunch with my big fake pregnant belly. Everyone would congratulate me, and be kind to me, thinking I was pregnant. I also was acting pregnant on the show and feeling so much love for this new baby that was coming and my partner on the show…

One day, the wardrobe girl was giving me my clothes to change into. She gave me the normal bra I wore – but when I tried to put it on, I could not fit in it.

"Your breasts have grown a whole new size! This is a C cup and I think you need a D cup now!" She was amazed.

She got me a new D cup bra. It fit perfectly.

I felt so shocked. But because I had studied psychobiology in college, it all made sense.

I had the baby on the show.

A few weeks later, when my body thought I was no longer pregnant, my breasts went back to their normal size.

Our bodies are so responsive to our thoughts!

Practice 39. Visualizing

Make sure your heart is wide open.

Do Practice 1, Heartfullness Meditation, to get you into that soft, receptive state. Make sure your heart feels full of love and joy.

Visualize what you want. Everyone has one or two sensory modalities that are strongest, so start with that modality. For example, I feel very strong emotions and very strong body sensations (kinesthetic), so I usually start with how something *feels* both emotionally and then physically. You may be more visual or auditory, so start there and then allow the rest to fill in. Don't force it. Visualization should feel effortless and fun.

Do the below list in the order of what's the easiest and richest feeling for you.

- Feel it as if it is here.
- Feel the emotions of it.
- Allow yourself to see it.
- Allow yourself to hear it.
- Allow yourself to discern the fragrance of it (if that's appropriate).
- Allow yourself to touch it and to discern the physical feeling of it, the texture, the temperature, the hard or softness of it, the weight of it, etc.
- Allow yourself to taste it (if that's appropriate!).

Visualize it in as many senses as you can so that you feel even better now, so that you feel immersed in this thing you desire, in this moment. Visualize it so it feels as real as it can, just for the pleasure of visualizing. Note the emotions you feel. Make that emotional state your new emotional state. Live in the feeling of your vision being manifest.

And keep visualizing it as many times a day as you wish, but don't look to see if it has manifested or not. Simply visualize it so that you feel better in this moment. Use it only to feel amazing now. Don't visualize to make anything happen. Visualize because it feels so wonderful!

Let the Universe do the work and surprise you with what comes. Let the Universe surprise you when it comes. It'll be much better than what you visualize if you stay in that place of love.

Driving in Flow

One of the things that a lot of people are not conscious of is how they feel when they drive. I hear many people have negative beliefs about driving and I used to have it too. Any stress you have, even if it's about something like driving, affects your body in a negative way. The more relaxed and easy you are, the better your body will feel.

I was born in Los Angeles and have lived in Los Angeles most of my life. (I have lived in Hawaii, and New York and for a summer in Montana as well.)

I have driven here most of my life. I used to always be late. It felt so embarrassing to be late so much of the time and it did not feel good for my relationships.

Then I realized that I had a belief about myself that 'I am always late.' I realized that was not a relevant belief, so I quickly started to find new ways of thinking that I practiced until they became my truth. Now, I get around Los Angeles quicker, easier, and more effortlessly than ever.

I have been practicing a few things to allow me to do this.

But first, just to see the difference, my dear, brilliant, and talented friend Julie Richardson came back into Los Angeles. She had worked here for a few years, and she had hated driving here. But for the last few years, she has been traveling all over the world and working in Vegas. (She produces amazing live burlesque circus shows!) She was staying with me this time, so when we went places, I would drive. She used to drive in Los Angeles near where I live now.

She felt amazed. She could not believe how empty the streets were for me as I drove. I got everywhere so easily and effortlessly and quickly. She marveled at how easy it was.

You can do this, too.

The way I have done this is that I focus on flowing to all I want.

I focus on everything being easy and effortless. My path is made clear for me. I flow through Los Angeles or wherever I am.

I never use that Tr (affic) word. That condition does not exist in my consciousness. When other people mention it, I silently thank the Universe that I flow to all I desire.

Then I simply talk to myself about how I love to flow, I say things like:

"I love getting where I want to go intuitively. I love getting where I want to go early or on time. I love arriving in a relaxed and easy and present way. It feels wonderful to arrive early. It feels beautiful to flow easily and effortlessly to all I desire. I feel delighted driving on empty streets all the time. I love driving in total effortless flow. It feels so fun for my way to be made clear. And it feels beautiful to love every driver, every car, every street, the trees, the beautiful houses, the wonderful people and dogs walking on the sidewalks. I feel in love with everyone. I feel everyone is perfect and beautiful."

I practiced thinking like this for several months. I was not trying to make anything happen. It just felt good to focus like this. It felt good to keep my heart flowing love to all on my path. It felt good to see the beauty everywhere I went.

If I do encounter anything unwanted, I relax, I practice loving everyone even more. I feel so thankful that I am arriving at the perfect time. I trust the perfection of it all. In fact, one of the few times I was late was when I was supposed to meet a business friend at my house and he was going to drive us to dinner, but I was so late driving home that we arranged to meet at the restaurant instead.

Once we started our dinner, he began to drink. He had several drinks. I feel much better being driven by sober people, especially because the only way to get to my house is a one lane road with a cliff on one side! At that moment, I felt so thankful for the fact that I had been so delayed that I had to meet him at the restaurant. The Universe knows that I love being driven by safe, sober people, and it knew his desire to drink (I had never seen him drink before so it was unknown to me!) I felt so thankful to drive myself home in a safe and sober way after dinner. And I felt so happy that I could love this man as he was drinking, knowing his perfection.

The more I practiced this, the more I found myself guided to turn this way or that, onto streets that were totally empty even when parallel streets were filled with other cars going the same direction as me. Now it feels amazing that so many times, I have left my house twenty minutes late and yet arrived ten minutes early. It feels so wonderful following the intuitions that guide me as I drive. Now, I drive in total flow all over Los Angeles. I feel love for everything and everyone. I feel delighted to arrive on time or early… I feel trust that whatever time I arrive will be perfect.

One time I was guided to drive a new way. I had never been on that street, and I was not sure how I would get where I was going from that street… then I saw *a castle*. It had a moat. It had turrets. It had a drawbridge and a large arched front door… It was a real castle in Los Angeles that I had never known existed. I knew in that moment that that's why I was sent down that street. And of course, I found myself inspired to the next street that was right for me to arrive at my destination on time… after I saw the castle!

This is letting the Universe work for me. You can do this in any area of your life.

Practice 40. Letting the Universe Guide Your Flow

Become aware if you have any beliefs about yourself, where you live, other drivers, that would feel good to be more in flow, that could feel even better.

Once you have identified those unaligned thoughts, do Practice 1, Heartfullness Meditation, to open your heart and to bring your mind and body into a deeper relaxation. When you feel open and full of love, from your soft, open heart, ask your genius Inner Being what would be a more fun way to think about this subject.

Then simply practice the new aligned beliefs until they become true for you, until it feels like your heart is singing when you say them to yourself or another. Practice these new thoughts until you own them, until they are yours. Practice these thoughts until you are so excited to drive or go anywhere.

Then, pay attention to the subtle impulses that the Source within you will provide you. The more relaxed you are, the more you will feel these inner promptings. As your mind gets freer about driving, as you feel more relaxed about how you always arrive at the perfect time and it always feels easy for you, you will find yourself flowing easily to all you desire. The UNIVERSE LOVES TO DO YOUR WORK! And the more you let the Universe do your work, the greater energy and pleasure you will have!

Synchronicities

Anytime you want to increase something, give it appreciation and recognition. (But don't appreciate them to make them increase, appreciate them because it feels so good to be have synchronicities and to be thankful!)

I feel so excited when I get synchronicities. I just love them! I keep a note in my phone that I can record any synchronicities that come to me. (I feel appreciation for Deepak who taught me this, decades ago! Thanks, D!) Whenever any synchronicity occurs, I make a record of it and then I say after the description how it made me feel and then I express my appreciation. For example, this is how I wrote one today:

> *"I was talking to a friend about Japan, and I remembered when I went there for the first time when I was 21. I remembered how fun it had been to go there to do a commercial. I felt the desire to see the commercial again. I did nothing. 2 days later, my friend, Teness, contacted me for the first time in years. She sent me a picture of me in that commercial! I had not told her or anyone about it. I posted the pic on Facebook. The next day, a friend from Japan posted the YouTube video of that commercial from YouTube in Japan! That*

feels so fun and perfect! I feel more connected to Peter Tramm, who was in the commercial with me and who is now a non-fizzie! I feel like clapping and laughing! Thank you! I love you!"

Here's another:

"I got an email from We are Laurel Canyon that there was a fire in my canyon. I thought I should email my neighbors and pack a bag but IB, you said 'nope, all is well, go meditate and write'... When I was meditating, the helicopters were very loud, but they did not bother me. By the time I was finished meditating there was silence. I checked the LAFD website and the fire was contained and cleared within another few minutes. The fire was totally put out. Thank me. I love me. I feel so thankful. That feels beautiful, it feels easy, it feels fun. I feel so secure. I feel so happy. Thank you, I love you! Thank me, I love me."

I could go on and on with the very long list of synchronicities that have happened and I try to record them as soon as they happen. I often re-read them when I arrive early to an appointment. The more I focus on them the more they increase. It's only 11 a.m. here as I write and already, I have had four synchronicities this morning. That feels soooo fun. It feels like the Universe is doing excellent work for me.

Practice 41. Being a Synchronicity Magnet

Get a notebook or go to the note section on your phone or computer.

Write down every synchronicity that happens, whether it's a tiny one or a big one. The more you value even the tiniest synchronicities, the more you will experience all of them.

Write out how you feel in the moment after you have written it and after receiving that synchronicity. Really feel the feelings in your heart, your gut, your whole body.

Write out your appreciation. Write it to whatever you believe in (God, Buddha, Mohammed, Allah, Jesus, the Universe, Love, yourself, etc.) then thank yourself for being open to them for being receptive, for being aware. Again, do this only because it feels so wonderful, not to make anything happen.

Chronic Pleasure

As I started to experience more pleasure in my body, I felt inspired to keep growing my pleasure. I did the same thing I did with synchronicities and improvements.

Almost anytime I felt pleasure, I make a note of it and put it in my phone or computer or just recognized it mentally and appreciated it. I kept a running list of pleasurable sensations, experiences, emotions.

That focus has become a pleasure in itself and it has enhanced my receptivity to pleasure. I did this until I felt immersed in pleasure, saturated in pleasure all day every day. Now my life feels drenched in pleasure. I feel immersed in pleasure.

Now the pleasure is so chronic, I simply experience it and feel thankful to it.

Even as I write, I am writing in great posture which feels wonderful, I feel beautiful pulses and contractions and waves of pleasure moving up my body as I write. My heart feels totally full of love and I feel sweet tears of love for you as I write… it feels sublime and I feel incredibly happy and thankful. I feel my whole-body buzzing with joy and electricity. When I drink water, I feel the water caressing my tongue and lips and throat as it goes down and it feels so sensuously pleasurable that I often catch myself moaning outloud, after a drink of water! Giggle!

If I do experience anything that is painful, I immediately relax deeper, I breathe into that area, I feel my heart open more so I can send love and adoration to that part. I ask my Inner Being to massage that part. I physically feel that gentle soothing massage penetrating any painful places and relaxing them deeper.

And then I follow my inspirations that lead me to letting it go or taking the appropriate action. I have trained myself to know that every sensation is bringing me more pleasure, so I stay relaxed and excited for the greater pleasure that is coming my way. Most pain in my life only lasts a few moments and then it vanishes.

Practice 42. Cultivating Chronic Pleasure

Keep a running list of all your pleasures. Anytime you feel great pleasure in any way, write out what it feels like as you experience it. (If you can, otherwise make a mental note. For example, driving feels so orgasmic for me most of the time, but I do not write it down, because being a safe driver also feels very pleasurable! Same with sexual pleasure and so many other pleasures! These can all be just a conscious appreciation vs. writing!)

These can be musical pleasure, sexual pleasure, food pleasure, touch pleasure, pleasure from nature, pleasure from exercise, pleasure from working, pleasure from connecting with others, pleasure from sex, pleasure from petting your pet, pleasure from meditation, pleasure from doing art, pleasure from dance, pleasure from caring for someone…

Whatever type of pleasure you experience, make a note of it either in writing or in your awareness and describe it in a way that feels yummy to you. Then thank your Divine nature. And thank yourself.

You will get so much pleasure that you can no longer write any of it down or you will be always writing 24/7… *that's* how I live.

Do this only because it feels good to focus on pleasure in *this moment*! This moment is all that matters.

In these ways, you are allowing the Universe to do the work. You are clearly expressing what you love in the form of appreciation and repeated focus and you are getting out of the way by appreciating all the magic in your life so that your Inner Being and the Universe and your body can do their genius work on your behalf. The Universe *loves* to do the work for you!

Chapter 11

Obstacles

I have offered so many practices and I know it may feel daunting. It may feel like it's impossible to purify everything, to stop negative thoughts, and harmful patterns, and it's totally fine if you feel that way. I felt that too, at the beginning. I had always been told the brain was complicated, that we had too much subconscious programming to ever be pure… but all that has changed within me, and within many of my clients. My mind feels completely transformed. It feels tranquil, receptive, and full of thankfulness, joy and love, so I know it can shift for you too.

Harnessing the Power of Obsession

I was in the shower one day, repeating this endless loop of how angry I was about something (I forget what it was now!) and I realized I was obsessed in a negative way. This felt totally hopeless.

After my shower I meditated so I could quiet that obsessive voice. Then I heard my Inner Brilliance say to me,

'Obsession itself is a neutral vehicle. You and most people have used it unconsciously to destroy yourselves and your lives, but you can use it in a new way. You can harness the repetitive action of the brain and use it for focusing on what you want.'

I felt my whole body radiating with thrill as I heard that. I felt a new power, a new lightness. I had no idea *how* to do it, but I loved that it could be done.

Over the next few hours and days, I felt so compelled to repeat certain phrases over and over.

I had heard about the practice of Japa, a Sanskrit word that meant to repeat a sacred name or phrase over and over and over all throughout the day. I began to say this sacred phrase as if it was Japa: "Thank you, Universe. I love you, Universe." I thought this with every step, every breath.

I felt it in my heart, opening my heart more. I said it silently from my soft, open heart, to every person I saw or heard about. I said it to every animal, every vegetable, every bit of food, every drink of water, every tree, every piece of furniture, every star and cloud and to the sun and the moon... "Thank you, Universe. I love you, Universe."

I felt so full of appreciation as I did it that it felt addictive. I feel addicted to appreciating everything. I feel addicted to seeing the Divine in everything. I did this day after day, all day every day.

After doing this for some time, I felt like I was listening to my brain say that instead of me thinking it. It felt like I had harnessed the power of obsession and now my brain was whispering "Thank you, Universe. I love you, Universe" to me day and night.

I have practiced Japa with lots of different sacred phrases. For example, "I am love."

"I am pure freedom." "I am light." And now my amazing, obsessive brain is obsessed with reminding me of these truths. This makes shifting your thoughts easier. The more you let your brilliant brain do the work, the better your body will feel.

Practice 43. Harnessing the Vehicle of Obsession for Your Benefit.

Determine your own sacred phrase that would feel good to say in a Japa way. It can be anything that lifts you up and lightens you.

Say it with every step, every breath until your brain is repeating it automatically.

If you make the intention, this will start to repeat itself when you need it; for example, if someone is talking about something negative or you see negative news, often your Inner Being will inspire you to say Japa on the sacred phrases you have practiced.

Using Music to Harness Obsession

You know how a song will get in your head and you will hear a phrase from it over and over? Often times many of us are not cognizant of the vibration of the lyrics we repeat over and over, so you want to find lyrics that really resonate with what you want. Using music is another way to harness obsession when you use it in a way that feels fabulous.

I listened to a bunch of songs and I picked just a phrase or two and I sing them to myself over and over. I make up aligned lyrics if the song lyrics go into resistance. If it's a catchy melody, I may use my own words but sing to that melody. You can do this with any songs that lift you up and lighten you. Make the song specific to you by shifting any lyrics so that the song feels in total flow for you.

Practice 44. Harnessing Obsession through Music

Because music has such an addictive power to it, I feel so excited for you to find songs that really lift you up and lighten you. Sing them or a part of them silently or out loud until they become an automatic part of your thinking.

You can pick any song or lyrics that you want (or make them up in your favorite rhythm) to bring more automatic joy into your life. Sing it until you are singing it with no effort, and it is just repeating itself in your head. Allow yourself to get obsessed with catchy lyrics and rhythms that really lift you up and lighten you and makes your heart sing!

But again, don't do anything to change your life. Do it because it feels good now. And as it feels good now, just keep repeating that aligned, happy phrase or that song over and over until you feel it is part of you, then your beautiful, loving brain will start repeating it for you.

What If the Pain Is Still There?

Does it feel like you have tried some of the exercises but it's not working? Do you feel frustrated or afraid it won't work for you? Or that this is too much work for you? Or do you feel like your case is something different?

I am not a doctor, I can only speak from what I have experienced and understand because of it, so again, check with your doctor before this.

For me, I was doing each of these exercises sort of naturally, meaning I did spend time every morning meditating and then writing out appreciation or my dreams or my improvements or synchronicities each morning. And then while I worked or drove or cooked, I was either keeping my attention on my heart and feeling the love there, or mentally practicing these tools – so it has all felt effortless – but in reality, I was practicing almost constantly. My biggest desire is to be in alignment with my Inner Being, so I just practiced these good feeling exercises and I HAD NO ATTACHMENT TO THE OUTCOME. I visualized what I wanted so it felt good now.

I feel love for my body, so it feels good now.

And any time I was measuring to see if something was better as opposed to appreciating it, some of the improvements I had been seeing would slip away… I found it so essential to only appreciate the improvements but not try to make things improve. That's such a fun balancing trick!

Here's an example of how I used these tools before I even knew them.

I had a melanoma on my face. My dermatologist had made an appointment with me to get it removed the following Tuesday. The Friday before, I was in my Whole Foods Market when I ran into a doctor I knew socially – he was dating my friend and we had all had a group dinner just a few months before. He said, "You have a melanoma!"

"Yes, I am getting it removed Tuesday."

He was alarmed, "You can't wait that long, you need to get it removed right away. Come to my office tomorrow morning. I will take care of it for you."

He gave me his card and we hugged goodbye.

I did not know the Law of Attraction at that time. But I had been meditating for almost a couple of decades by then. I felt scared. I wanted my skin to be smooth. I wanted my skin to be healthy. When I went home, I went into meditation. I meditated on the feeling of beauty, I see beauty in all of nature and in each person, so I knew it must be important to the Universe in some way.

I meditated not to cure my body, but to soothe myself from the fear that had come up when he told me I couldn't wait that long, and the fear of having my face cut. I kept meditating that day because the meditation on beauty felt wonderful. I intuitively did not want to focus on what was going on in my body. I meditated all that day and any time I woke up in the night, I meditated on that soothing feeling of beauty.

When I got up in the morning, my face was totally clear. There was no sign I had had any issue. I felt amazed and called the doctor.

"It's gone."

"What do you mean it's gone? That's impossible!"

"It's not there. There's no sign of it, it completely disappeared."

"I don't believe you, come in anyway!"

"…Okay."

The moment I walked into his office he looked at me and said, "I've never seen anything like that before in my life!"

He went on and on about how it was impossible. Yet it happened. *Everything you want that is right for you is possible!*

This is an example of the purity of my intention, even though this happened before I even heard of the Law of Attraction. This is an example of how I had no attachment to the outcome, I was simply tuning to a much better feeling so that I could soothe myself in that moment.

Find anything you can to feel better. Pleasure is the antidote to pain.

Practice 45. Letting Go of Any Outcome

Keep an awareness of yourself and a discernment so you can feel if you are 'trying, efforting, pushing,' or making any real effort to get what you want. If you keep letting those things go, you will keep relaxing. Focus on the idea that you are only doing anything to feel good in this moment. You are not trying to make anything happen. You are instead getting into a place of joy and letting that joy flow you to whatever you desire. You can also play with whatever sacred phrases or song lyrics you picked. As you keep relaxing and feeling as good as you can emotionally in this moment you will gradually become more in a state of pure *being*. This will be automatic. You will have harnessed the vehicle of obsession for your benefit. You will be in a state of being fully present and full of love. You will feel pure and innocent. And your body will thank you. Your body loves when you are pure being. Your body loves when you feel full of love.

Self-Soothing

One of the things that is so harmful to our bodies and our lives is to beat ourselves up if we are feeling something negative or if something unwanted is showing up. That compounds the problem.

When I had the incessant fatigue, I would get so mad at myself every time I felt tired. This aggravated the issue. Now I felt tired *and* angry. My inability to stay awake increased each time I did that.

The antidote is to approve of yourself and to approve of whatever is happening and to practice soothing yourself.

When I learned to soothe myself, even with my resistance or my needing a nap, my fatigue gradually diminished. Narcolepsy became such a gift to me because it trained me that I needed to be soothing and kind to myself and to others. It made me more understanding, more loving, more gentle, than I had even known was possible, with myself and with you.

Learning self-soothing is really one of the best skills anyone can learn. (I wish we taught it in every grade in schools!) It's a lifelong practice of being kind and gentle and loving to yourself. It's the practice of accepting yourself where you are and giving approval to yourself where you are, while you are also turning it around so that whatever the situation, circumstance, or person is, you are allowing that situation, person, or circumstance to benefit you, to be a gift to you.

For example: let's say you feel tired...

First, find a place to lie down when you can, where it is safe and comfortable. Then start telling yourself that this is a perfect time to take a nap. It feels wonderful to take a nap. It's okay to feel tired. You deserve this nap. This nap will benefit you, prosper you, and make you healthier. You feel so happy to take this nap and then wake up feeling so wonderful...

And in that way, give yourself the soothing that you need.

If something unwanted comes, again, don't push against it, don't beat yourself up, instead just say something like, *"This person, experience, condition, or situation is such a gift to me, I may not know yet how it's gifting me, but I feel so excited to find out. This is benefitting me, prospering me, and making my body full of more pleasure and more energy. I know this is really leading me to all I really want. I feel so secure and safe in knowing that this is leading me to all I desire."*

You can literally make it up the way you want it to be. Everything that happens to you is a divine gift. *It actually is leading you to all you desire* – if you don't resist it. And since our bodies and the world are a reflection of our thoughts, emotions, and actions, as you soothe yourself, you are actually also raising your vibration on that subject so more of what is wanted will come to you. Although, remember the paradox: only raise your vibration on that subject so that you feel good *now*!

Practice 46. Self-Soothing

Practice being kind, gentle, approving, and accepting of yourself, especially when you are feeling resistance, fatigue, or pain. Let yourself know that however you feel, you are loved, and you are being ben-efitted and prospered by it. See if you can feel thankful for the fatigue or pain or emotional upset because it's inspiring you to be more loving with yourself, which will benefit you and all your relationships. It's bringing you more pleasure and more energy even if you don't yet know how it's doing that. Any time you are kind to yourself, applaud yourself. Celebrate yourself for your own kindness. You will find your body thrives on self-soothing.

What If the Pain or Fatigue Is Still There?

I know everybody is different, so the more you are in alignment with your Inner Being, the more you will be intuitively guided for what works best for you.

And I feel happy to share a few things that worked for me, in case this spurs your inspiration. You are welcome to try any or to find your own path.

Practices I Feel Are Amazing that You May Enjoy:

Wim Hof Method:

I have been doing the Wim Hof method for only about a year, as of this writing. Wim uses a certain kind of intense breathing with breath holding and cold water exposure that helps your body deal with stress, cold, and inflammation and so much more. I was already in Chronic Pleasure and had great energy when I started it, but I *love* doing it because I can feel it is giving me more pleasure and more energy and greater endurance. Many of his classes talk about how it can reduce inflammation, reduce stress, increase stamina and endurance, and reduce pain. I don't get any inflammation, stress, or pain so I don't have personal experience that it does that, but it has provided me more energy and stamina and made me much more comfortable in the cold. It has increased my lung capacity too.

I have read a lot of testimonials from people saying it has helped diminish their pain.

If this feels intriguing to you, you may want to check it out. I do it almost every morning and I really enjoy the whole practice. There is a free app with the first three lessons on it. It's called The Wim Hof Method and if you like the first three classes, then you may like the Fundamentals course, which I took. I think it may have ten or twelve classes. I used to hate cold water, but I recently went swimming in the high arctic in four degrees Celsius and I was totally relaxed and enjoyed the whole experience. And now I love taking a cold shower at the end of my warmer shower. I feel thankful to Wim for his instruction in this! Plus, Wim is in pure love. He is pure light and totally inspiring! I love him!

The Egoscue Method

A lot of pain and fatigue can come from improper posture. Pete Egoscue recognized this and he devised exercises that help people activate muscles that have been dormant and help muscles that have been compensating to relax. You can find videos on the internet to see more about it or you can go to a clinic or have a Skype appointment with a therapist.

I *love* the Egoscue method because it has been so helpful to me. Before I knew the Law of Attraction, I had a shoulder injury. I had been going to physical therapy for about six months and I was still in pain. I could not even carry my purse on that side, nor dance, do yoga, or even walk while swinging my arms without pain.

When I was dealing with this long-term shoulder injury, a friend told me about the Egoscue Method. She just said I should try it and that it was super helpful. She said Pete Egoscue was helping athletes by helping them have better function of their bodies.

I went to the first appointment I could get. They actually gave me exercises to make my hips straight rather than anything for my shoulders. I did the exercises that day when I got home, I did them again the next day and then the third day, I flew to Australia and I did them in the morning that day as well. Deepak Chopra and I are friends, we had had dinner that night and he had invited me to his workshop the next day, so I went to his workshop the next day after doing the Egoscue exercises in the morning. This was the fourth day after my first Egoscue appointment. My shoulder was feeling better already…

After the workshop, I had the urge to get on this public trampoline that had people who were spotting the bouncers and safety belts (I love that Australia has so many fun things to play on!).

I got on and started bouncing. I heard my Inner Knowing tell me to do a backflip… a backflip requires that I throw my arms back and I was concerned about my shoulder. I said to my Inner Knowing that I did not want to do a backflip. I felt my Inner Knowing insisting I do one, so I did a backflip. It actually felt fine, so I did a few more.

Then my Inner Knowing directed me to do a double backflip. I was in safety lines, so I knew it was safe, except that you have to throw your arms back harder to do a double. I resisted it for a few moments, but I felt the Inner Knowing within me being so insistent, so I threw a double backflip.

It felt fine… then I felt my Inner Knowing directing me to throw a triple backflip. I had never done a triple backflip even in safety lines, so I felt wary. I also knew I would really have to throw my arms back very hard to rotate fast and small enough to do a triple. I felt my Inner Knowing being insistent. I threw a triple backflip.

I heard a pop. The girl spotting me heard the pop, too. I stopped bouncing. I could feel my shoulder was different. I got off the trampoline and sat on the bench to just feel what was happening… I realized my shoulder had been popped back into place. It felt amazing! The Egoscue method had strengthened the muscles enough that needed to be strengthened and relaxed the muscles that were compensating enough so that my shoulder could get into place, and the triple back had moved it into the perfect position to pop it into place. I tested the feeling in my shoulder for a few more minutes and it felt totally normal. I went back on the trampoline for another round. Everything felt wonderful! I then walked back to my hotel swinging my arms, carrying my purse and feeling so excited. I did the Egoscue exercises again that night and my shoulder kept feeling better and better. Within two more days I was dancing salsa again and doing yoga again. And Egoscue has helped me with lots of other things. You can find them online or maybe in your city. You can also do appointments via Skype if there are no clinics in your area.

Example of Egoscue on Kyphosis:

A friend of mine had severe kyphosis (hunchback) and it had been going on for years. I told him about Egoscue. I saw him after he had had five Egoscue sessions… his back was totally straight and aligned. He looked so much better! He was beaming. I felt amazed at how quickly his body had shifted. It felt miraculous. He said he was out of pain and feeling so much better and he was going to keep going to make sure to strengthen the new muscles that were keeping him more upright.

Products I Feel Benefit My Body and May Feel Fun for You to Try

Fascia Blaster and/ or the Gua Sha and The Fascianator:

The fascia blaster, The Fascianator, and the gua sha soften fascia that has become stiff. Fascia is the largest organ in your body and the biggest sensory organ and the organ that holds the most toxins. Fascia is in and around every muscle, every joint, in your brain, around your blood vessels and your nerves… it's everywhere!

I got the fascia blaster (fasciablaster.com) to deal with my calves, which got tight when I danced. But then, I realized how my entire fascia throughout my body *loved* being made more supple by this funny tool.

Now I fascia-blast or use the gua sha or the Fascianator on different parts of my body daily, and it keeps my body feeling supple, pliable, and soft.

I had had an injury on my back when I was eighteen that was still in my body. It felt like sharp shards of glass were all along my spine. I asked my amazing friend and masseuse, Joey Calderon to use the fascia blaster and gua sha between my rib bones on my back and up and down my spine. After a few sessions my whole spine became more soft, flexible, and supple. All the sharpness disappeared. My back feels fluid and amazing now. I also occasionally get marathon fascia blasting sessions on my whole body from Joey Calderon. Our record so far of him fascia blasting and using the gua sha on my whole body is six hours straight… *talk about ecstatic pleasure*!!! I feel so appreciative that he is an athlete, so he has the stamina and endurance to do it. When we do those marathons, I feel so high, I feel totally intoxicated by the suppleness of my fascia. It feels like so much energy is streaming through me.

Freeing my fascia has provided me more energy and more pleasure. Even after the sessions, my fascia is more supple for a while and the more soft and relaxed the fascia is, the more I can perceive pleasure.

I never had cellulite but the fascia blaster also does break up fat and cellulite, if that appeals to you.

If you can get someone to do your whole body or back side (you can do your front side pretty easily), it would feel *amazing*! Whenever Joey comes to work on me, within a few minutes of him fascia blasting or using the gua sha on any part of my body I feel streaming energy flowing through me and I feel so high… it feels incredible.

Just so you know, it may not feel that good at first. Joey said that most people can only take the gua sha or the fascia blaster for a few minutes to start. As you begin to break up tight fascia it can feel painful – if it does, simply back off, either use feather-light pressure or stop in that area… over time you will find your fascia becoming more supple. But for me, it always felt good.

I got the gua sha to see if it felt good over scar tissue. Not only did it diminish my scar tissue, but it's made my hands more supple and more beautiful! And it took away some hand wrinkles! (You gotta love that!)

And I use it on my face and my under-eye wrinkles and forehead wrinkles mostly disappeared. I also use it on the inside of my jaw muscles. They are becoming so soft and relaxed with daily use of the gua sha.

I had used it before I had watched the instructional videos, so I just followed my inspiration on how to use it… well, for me, the way I use it is totally different than the way those instructional videos show how to use it. But it has really worked for me! I am ridiculously fast and use quite a bit of pressure with it on my face – even under and above my eyes – but my whole face and hands feel and look so much better… That's why I suggest you want to follow your own inner guidance as much as you can.

The Fascianator is also helping to keep my fascia supple. I use it most days. It's a hard, small in diameter roller that can really soften the tissue. I have become more flexible after using it and can now do some stretches I could never do before in my life! That feels sooooo wonderful!

The Bob

I also got this device called The Bob. It's a calf stretcher and strengthener and I love it. As you bob on it, it strengthens and stretches all the muscles around your ankles so that your ankles, feet, and calves all become stronger and more flexible (http://exercisebob.com/).

It's strengthening all the muscles in my ankles and calves in a balanced way so that they all work better. My feet feel more connected to the earth. It's supposed to help with plantar fasciitis, which I don't have. I just wanted to try it because it looked fun, and it is fun, and it feels wonderful!

Yoga Trapeze!

I have a yoga trapeze, which hangs from some beams in my living room and that I use often to really stretch my body and my fascia. It feels incredible and it stretches my body in ways nothing else seems able to do. I can also go upside down in it and it holds me upside down in a relaxed way. I always feel so much better after I use it. I feel thankful to my dear, beautiful, loving friend, Courtney Fenton, who recommended it to me because she knew I would love it!

Raw Organic Cacao Butter and Raw Organic Cacao Powder

First, this tastes amazing. Also, both of these substances contain anandamide. Ananda is the Sanskrit word for bliss. Anandamide is the neurotransmitter we have in our bodies and brains that gives us that feeling of bliss.

I have been drinking the raw organic cacao powder with purified water, coconut oil, and stevia to make a chocolate milk type drink for a while and it tastes yummy, provides good brain food in the coconut oil, the cacao is a superfood, and it provides anandamide, polyphenols, vitamins and minerals, and antioxidants. Cacao has a lot of magnesium too, which can be good for muscles that *love* to work out (like mine!). Plus, the body uses magnesium in so many essential processes and many people would benefit from ingesting more of it.

I also use the cacao butter to make sugar-free deserts and to use as a body moisturizer and a lip gloss that smells like chocolate… YUM!

Drs. Moskowitz and Golden in their workbook *Neuroplastic Transformation* said, *"Anandamide is synthesized and released at synapses, blocking inflammation, shutting off Long Term Potentiation, Reverting Microglia…. Anandamide acts both as a neurotransmitter and immune system regulator. It works on the cannabinoid receptors in the brain, the same receptors activated by marijuana. These receptors serve multiple functions and are extremely varied in and important in soothing, stopping inflammation, stimulating appetite, controlling nausea, regulating emotions, controlling pain and activating pleasure circuits. Anandamide also... tells the nucleus of the nerve cell to change the way its DNA promotes inflammation and cell death."*[4]

That means anandamide is super good for you!

I had been using the cacao as food and on my body (it smells like chocolate) before I read this, and I felt so thrilled that I had intuitively done something again that enhances my health and well-being. The anandamide will pass into your blood stream if you use the raw organic cacao butter on your skin. Just make sure to blot yourself before you get dressed so you don't stain your clothes! It's pretty oily. It smells amazing, but the scent does not last.

sota.com

Sota makes these devices that are meant to provide greater well-being to the body. I felt healthy already, but I got three health products just to see how healthy I could be...

I feel so *amazed*! I got these three health products that really ramp up my energy and my life force. One unit sends microcurrents of electricity through the pulse points on my wrist (the silver pulser) and another unit creates the same microcurrents except it goes to site-specific places in the rest of my body in the deeper tissues (the magnetic pulser). Another unit helps with keeping the emotions happy, calm, and relaxed (the bio tuner). I am already happy, so I just got that last one to see if it makes me even happier, and because I wondered if it would feel beneficial to others, and so far, I see it is benefitting me. More on that below. These three products all seem to work together very well.

I have been using the silver pulser and the magnetic pulser for about a year. I am so excited about the benefits I am receiving! The effects seem to be cumulative.

---

4   Moskowitz, Michael H., and Marla DePolo Golden. *Neuroplastic Transformation Workbook*. 1st ed. Neuroplastic Partners, LLC, 2013.

When I first started using them, I detoxed a bit. I was more tired than normal. Now I have been feeling more and more energy. My energy feels *amazing*! My body feels so healthy and strong and energized. I am feeling much more energy and am not very sore after I work out (even when I am working out twice as much as before). That's huge for me. I have tried so many things to soothe my muscles and get more energy before, including the Bemer and corydalis (a vitamin). So far, these Sota products soothe and energize my body in amazing ways.

This Canadian company is not allowed to make any health claims. I found videos on the internet that alerted me to these products and that totally inspired me to take back my power and try them just to see how fabulous I can feel. These instruments are promoting wellness and general health, well-being, and relaxation. These are Wellness Tools and Wellness Products just like meditation, exercise, good food, and being happy all support good health.

If you want to do your own research, you can buy them and return them if they are not right for you.

I bought these instruments with the intention of simply doing an experiment and doing my own research to see if I felt any better or not. I knew within a few days of using each of them, that these were *amazing* for me. My body feels better, even with working out almost every day. My sleep is improving, and my energy is far, far greater. My memory is increasing. My productivity is increasing. My ability to take care of things easily is increasing. And my skin looks better! (YAY!)

A Fun Example of the Power of Alignment:

I had a client who contacted me via FaceTime because she had food poisoning. We had worked together in the past, but she wanted to work with me in that moment and fortunately I had time. She said she had had dinner with a friend when she had become nauseous and had to be taken home. I asked her how she felt about this friend. She said she felt awkward, and afraid that he liked her much more than she liked him. She felt like she wanted to escape from his oppressive energy. He seemed so possessive of her and she just wanted to be friends. Once she told me, I gave her a suggestion. I asked her to write out what she wanted to feel. I told her to write out all the qualities of Source and ascribe them to herself and then ascribe the qualities of Source to him. She did it while we were on FaceTime together.

Within a few moments her nausea had gone away. She looked radiant and relaxed. She could not believe how quickly her body had let it go. She changed her thoughts and her body shifted.

More Evidence of the Power of Alignment

My client had kidney stones. His doctor had told him he needed surgery. He was terrified of surgery. I calmed him down, I gave him the suggestion that the stones would dissolve and pass through him easily. He was on the way to get the surgery when he passed the kidney stones in the cab! He was amazed. The doctor was amazed. It had hurt a bit, but he did not have to have surgery and it had happened so effortlessly and automatically. He sent me a big bouquet of flowers... I love my job!

Another Example of the Power of Alignment!

A girl I coached had been wanting to stop drinking. She felt it was getting in the way of her life. She also had a terrible skin condition that was really uncomfortable for her. Through deep relaxation, I helped her release some blocks she had about a few things growing up and she has not had a drink since. Within a week her skin cleared up.

Your body is a reflection of your thoughts, emotions, and actions. If you can gently do any of the Practices in this book, and do them consistently with no sense of obligation, no sense of trying to fix anything and only a sense of doing this for fun, because it feels good, then you cannot help but be benefitted.

I feel so much love for you. I want you to feel the bliss, the chronic pleasure, the vibrant energy that you were born to feel. You deserve to feel *wonderful* all the time.

One Last Thing

Sometimes, people feel sick because they have a lifelong dream that they are not following. If you have tried everything in this book, and you still feel fatigue or pain, it may be because you have a wonderful and exciting dream that wants to be birthed! Sometimes, ignoring the subtle inspirations that are guiding us to what we want, ignoring the inspirations that are leading us to our creations, can literally make us ill.

The answer then, is to follow every good-feeling inspiration. The answer is to become willing to do what you are being called to do. If you have been feeling called but have not heeded the call, now is the time to start. It's okay if you start now; you are starting at the perfect time. You have done everything in perfect time. You are right on track.

If that is the case, take a look at any actions that you feel inspired to take, or any desires or dreams you have that you have not allowed in yet. And ask the Source within you to guide you, to inspire you in that direction. Affirm that you are willing.

Make sure your heart is soft and open and full of love, then listen to the inspirations that come. Even as you start moving in the direction of your calling, your dreams, your desires, you will feel better and better.

It's not like you have to make anything happen. Even if your dream feels big to you, relax, keep your heart wide open, full of love, keep your body and mind receptive to the genius within you and just follow each tiny step. If you don't know what to do, just welcome every inspiration, every intuition and let each one guide you to whatever is the next step. Your path is already laid out before you; simply keep following the next best feeling step and you will find yourself following your dreams and realizing your dreams, while you become more of the person you came here to be.

All of the practices in this book are designed to make you receptive to your inspirations and to allow yourself to flow with divine clarity. You cannot fail. You will succeed.

A thought for you:

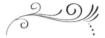

Love lives in you. You live in love.
Trust lives in you. You live in trust.
Answers live in you. You live in the answer.
Soulutions live in you. You live in soulutions.
My soul lives in you. You live in my soul.
Abundance lives in you. You live in abundance.
Fun lives in you. You live in fun.
Humor lives in you. You live in humor.
Laughter lives in you. You live in laughter.
Health lives in you. You live in health.
Pleasure lives in you. You live in pleasure.
Clarity lives in you. You live in clarity.
Infinite resources live in you. You live in infinite resources.
Infinity lives in you. You live in infinity.
Eternity lives in you. You live in eternity.
Fulfillment lives in you. You live in fulfillment.
Connection lives in you. You live in connection.
The Universe lives in you. You live in the Universe.
Bliss lives in you. You live in bliss.
By Karen Lorre

Chapter 12:

What You Learned

You are at the end of this book, but hopefully not the end of this practice. It would feel wonderful to let yourself be immersed in this book's wisdom and practices. Allow yourself to do the practices as often as you can, until you feel saturated in the perfect health, vibrant energy, and chronic pleasure that you deserve. If you do the practices that make you feel the best long enough, you will start to feel your bliss, your love, your pleasure, your energy, is automatic. You will be immersed in the pure being of who you are. Life will feel endlessly effortless.

As a reminder here are all the practices and what each one does.

Chapter 4: Applying the Solution

PRACTICE 1, HEARTFULLNESS MEDITATION. This opens your heart, relaxes your mind and body, and keeps you tranquil and in the flow. It's a great practice to do before many of the other practices.

PRACTICE 2, RELEVANT: FOCUSING ON WHAT LIFTS YOU UP AND LIGHTENS YOU. This helps you to understand whether whatever you are focused upon is serving you and the world or not.

PRACTICE 3, ABC SELF-LOVE GAME. This is a fun game that feels playful and light and truly enhances your sense of self-adoration. It's also fun to play with others for deeper connection.

PRACTICE 4, HAVE FUN FLIRTING WITH YOUR BODY. This fun practice feels so yummy and really promotes a deeper love for your amazing body.

Chapter 5: Learn to Allow Yourself to Feel Loved Easily

PRACTICE 5, PRACTICING FEELING APPROVED OF AND VALIDATED. This allows you to receive the approval and validation you need so you feel resourced and yummy and it now feels easy to flow that approval and validation out to others.

PRACTICE 6, PRACTICE FEELING UNDERSTOOD. This allows you to receive the understanding that you need so you feel resourced and understood and it now feels easy to flow that feeling of understanding out to others.

PRACTICE 7, FEELING ACCEPTED. This allows you to receive the acceptance you need so you feel resourced and accepted and it now feels easy to flow that feeling of acceptance out to others.

PRACTICE 8, ALLOWING THE UNIVERSE TO FEEL PROUD OF YOU. This allows you to receive the feeling of the Entire Universe being proud of you, so you feel resourced and proud of yourself and it now feels easy to flow the feeling of being proud to yourself and others.

PRACTICE 9, ALLOWING YOURSELF TO FEEL CELE-BRATED. This allows you to receive the celebration you enjoy or need, so you feel resourced and celebrated unconditionally and it now feels easy to flow that celebration out to others.

Chapter 6: Transforming Easily

PRACTICE 10, UPGRADE YOUR THOUGHTS ON ANY SUB-JECT. This allows you to feel a new fresh reality coming forth and to feel wonderful.

PRACTICE 11, BYPASS MY OWN PERSONALITY TO SEE THE BEST IN ME. This allows you to feel your divine nature easily.

PRACTICE 12, BYPASS THE PERSONALITY OF OTHERS TO SEE THE BEST IN THEM. This allows you to see the divinity in others easily.

PRACTICE 13, COMPASSION, FEELING THE SAME AS SOURCE. This keeps you feeling wonderful no matter what's happening around you.

PRACTICE 14, EMPATHY WITH SOURCE This allows you to feel safe and happy no matter where you are or whom you are with.

Chapter 7: Changing Cultural Hypnotic Suggestions

PRACTICE 15, CREATING YOUR HI STORIES. This is a fun way to transmute the past, so it fuels you and enlivens your present and future.

PRACTICE 16, RELEASE ANY CULTURAL HYPNOTIC SUGGESTIONS THAT DON'T SERVE YOU. This is a fun way to see how you may have been programmed and to take back your power.

PRACTICE 17, RELEASE ANY GUARDING OR PROTECTION. This keeps you soft and relaxed and able to feel happier and healthier and enables you to attract more goodness of what you want.

PRACTICE 18, RELEASING ANY CULTURAL HYPNOSIS OF FOOD. This is a fun way to eat healthier.

PRACTICE 19, RELEASING NEGATIVE EMOTIONS THAT CAUSED ALLERGIES. This is a fun feeling way to feel good even when exposed to things that used to cause allergies. *Please check with your doctor before engaging with any allergens.*

PRACTICE 20, RELEASING THE CULTURAL HYPNOSIS OF AGING. This helps you tap into your ever-rejuvenated, eternal self.

PRACTICE 21, RELEASING CULTURAL HYPNOSIS OF ASTROLOGY. This gives you total freedom, connection to the Divine and power no matter what the stars, planets, and moons are doing.

PRACTICE 22, CREATE YOUR OWN HYPNOTIC SUGGES-TIONS. This allows you to thrive in any way that feels right for you.

Chapter 8: Pleasure Is the Antidote to Pain

PRACTICE 23, FINDING PLEASURES YOU CAN DO EASILY. This does just what it says. You find pleasures that are right for you and that feel easy to do.

PRACTICE 24, HARNESSING THE POWER OF BLIS-SIPLINE. This provides you a path to making everything easy and pleasurable.

PRACTICE 25, RELAXATION THROUGHOUT YOUR DAY. This helps you be more tranquil and more attuned to pleasure.

PRACTICE 26, RECEIVING INTERNAL CARESSES. This enables you to feel epic pleasure whenever you want.

PRACTICE 27, TURN ON This keeps your creative energies flowing and feels wonderful.

PRACTICE 28, TRANSMUTE PAST EXPERIENCES INTO JEWELS. This chapter helps you find the gifts in contrasting situations.

PRACTICE 29, APPRECIATING IMPROVEMENT. This feel-good practice causes you to recognize and nurture improvements.

Chapter 9: Your Eternal Self

PRACTICE 30, TRUSTING THE INSPIRATIONS YOU RECEIVE. Practice the secret to trusting your inspirations.

PRACTICE 31, CONNECTING TO NON-PHYSICAL ENERGY. An easy way to connect to those you love or would love to know.

PRACTICE 32, REAFFIRM YOUR ETERNAL AMAZING SELF. If you are ever feeling like you are an imposter or just not confident in who you are, do this.

PRACTICE 33, DISCOVER YOUR UNCONDITIONALLY ADORABLE NATURE. Discover how you are adored even when you don't feel it.

PRACTICE 34, EXPERIENCE YOUR INVINCIBLE NATURE. Discover how unstoppable and powerful you are.

Chapter 10: Letting the Universe Do the Work

Learn to relax and let the Universe carry you like on a magic carpet ride to all you desire.

PRACTICE 35, DEVELOPING INTUITION. How to discern real intuition from that which is not accurate and how to increase your ability to live intuitively.

PRACTICE 36, YOUR EVERY THOUGHT IS YOUR PRAYER. Get greater self-awareness and more power with your prayers.

PRACTICE 37, ASKING QUESTIONS THAT FEEL GOOD. Discover a fun way to get high naturally and stay in alignment.

PRACTICE 38, HEARTFULL AWARENESS THROUGH OUT YOUR DAY. This practice keeps you in love and in the flow.

PRACTICE 39, VISUALIZING. How to visualize in a way that really is effective and feels amazing.

PRACTICE 40, LETTING THE UNIVERSE GUIDE YOUR FLOW. How to stay out of the way and find what's best for you.

PRACTICE 41, BEING A SYNCHRONICITY MAGNET. How to increase your synchronicities so that your whole life feels magical.

PRACTICE 42, CULTIVATING CHRONIC PLEASURE. Pleasure is the antidote to pain. How to increase its frequency throughout your day.

Chapter 11: Obstacles:

PRACTICE 43, HARNESSING THE VEHICLE OF OBSESSION FOR YOUR BENEFIT. Learn how to let the obsessive quality of your mind work for you.

PRACTICE 44, HARNESSING OBSESSION THROUGH MUSIC. Let music take you to where you want to go.

PRACTICE 45, LETTING GO OF ANY OUTCOME. Allow yourself to feel fully satisfied now.

PRACTICE 46, SELF-SOOTHING. One of the most important skills that should be taught in every grade of school!

Remember to do each practice *because it feels good*, not to make anything happen.

My Desire for You:

My desire for you is that you feel inspired to do all that is written in this book and that you receive all the incredible, blissful pleasure and energy that I feel every day (or more!). I wish for you to feel free and joyful and able to do and to be and to have what you desire. I wish for you that your body feels how very lovable and perfect it is now and that it gets healthier, happier, more energized, and more pleasured. My wish for you is that you feel totally loved, totally resourced, and totally supported in all you do. I desire that you do these practices enough that you merge into that Pure Beingness of who you *Really Are.* That state where there is nothing you have to do, you are simply carried on a magic carpet to all you desire, you are following inspiration with effortless ease, while feeling vibrant energy and chronic, extraordinary pleasure.

What to Do Next:

After you have done each of these exercises a few times, find the combo of what works for you in each day. Keep practicing. There is tremendous benefit in consistent practice on a moment-to-moment basis.

Share your success and stay in touch.

Contact me with any questions or to share your experience at YummyMeditations.com or KarenLorre@me.com.

Acknowledgments

I feel deeply thankful to Dr. Deepak Chopra for his friendship and for teaching me how to meditate and so much more. I feel appreciation that he taught me so much about how the mind affects the body. I feel massive appreciation that he also taught me through his example how to exude pure love.

I feel so much love and appreciation for Dr. Bruce Lipton and his amazing partner, Margaret Horton, for their friendship and for all Bruce has taught me about epigenetics and for all that Margaret has taught me about life and partnership and friendship through her loving example.

I feel incredible appreciation for Jerry and Esther Hicks and Abraham for teaching me a few things that were essential to my healing and happiness.

I feel thankful to Silje Vallestad, and Future Talks who invited me on the invitation-only expedition to the high arctic with one hundred world thought leaders to discuss the future and who invited me to teach and lead meditations daily on the expedition boat. I feel thankful for all the amazing new friends I have from that trip. It feels epic!

I feel thankful to Angela Lauria, Cheyenne Giesecke, Bethany Davis, and all the wonderful people at the Author Incubator for making this a fun, easy project.

I feel thankful to my amazing business partner, Marc Mollicone, for his incredible genius wisdom and help and support!

I feel so thankful to my amazing mom who taught me to always be kind and to focus on the things I love in others. I feel so thankful that when I was little, my mom taught me how anytime I was sick, it was because I had something that was bothering me emotionally. I didn't like it at the time, but now, that clarity has improved my life in a huge way. I feel thankful to my loving Dad who came to me after he was non-physical and has been inspiring me ever since. I feel so much love for my brilliant brother, Greg, and his beautiful wife Gina, and their incredible kids: Macie, Tessa, and Cole. You all amaze me with your unique brilliance!

I feel so thankful to my wonderful friends, Shirley Solie and Goody Cable, who turned me on to the Science of Mind when I was so young.

I feel epic love for my friends, Carilyn Davidson and Norma Eckroate who play a fun mastermind game with me every day that allows me to share all my happiness with them and to share in their joys too. I feel so thankful for how we all support and inspire each other.

I feel thankful for the Morgan James Publishing team: Special thanks to David Hancock, CEO & Founder for believing in me and my message. To my Author Relations Manager, Bonnie Rauch, thanks for making the process seamless and easy. Many more thanks to everyone else, but especially Jim Howard, Bethany Marshall, and Nickcole Watkins.

I feel thankful to my many *amazing* clients who have shown me in each session just how powerfully our minds affect our bodies. Even when we don't do a session on the body, everyone tends to look ten or fifteen years younger and so much more beautiful after each session. That feels so thrilling each time I see it. I feel so much love and appreciation for you. I feel appreciation for all your wonderful questions that caused me to find wonderful solutions! I feel epic appreciation for you sharing with me how effortlessly you shift into what you are wanting. That lets me know my coaching is powerful, effective and *easy!*

I feel immense thankfulness to my all my inspiring and loving friends.

I feel so thankful to all the pain and suffering and fatigue I had, which inspired me to live in the pure pleasure and love and vibrant energy I now have. I feel thankful for all the contrast in my life, which has led me to live a magical life. I feel thankful to all the rascals in my life, who trained me to love unconditionally!

I feel the deepest, most profound love for my Inner Being, who guides me, loves me, pleasures me, and resources me completely in every moment.

Thank You!

I feel appreciation for you reading *Chronic Pleasure*! This is the beginning of a life-enhancing and delightful way of life. The fact that you've gotten to this point in the book helps me understand something beautiful about you: you are ready. You're ready to feel better emotionally and physically, than you ever have before.

After you have done each of these exercises a few times, find the combo of what works for you in each day. Keep practicing. There is tremendous benefit in consistent practice on a moment-to-moment basis.

To support you in feeling better emotionally and physically, I created the **FEELING FABULOUS ASSESSMENT** just for you. It's a simple diagnostic assessment to help you get crystal-clear about which areas you need to shift to feel fabulous emotionally and physically. You can get your copy of the **FEELING FABULOUS ASSESSMENT** at ChronicPleasureBook.com.

Share your success and stay in touch, or for more information email me at KarenLorre@me.com.

I feel passionate about you feeling as good as you can! You feeling awesome brings me some of my greatest joy.

About the Author

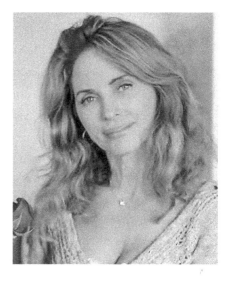

Karen Lorre studied psychobiology (how the mind affects the body) in college. She has had a lifelong interest in psychobiology, epigenetics, neuroscience, health, and spirituality. She has studied the Science of Mind since 1985, has been meditating consistently since 1991, and has studied the Law of Attraction since 2009. Throughout her life, Karen found she had a natural gift for receiving direct communication and downloads from the Infinite Loving Divine and intuitive clarity.

Karen is an actress and has done over a thousand hours of TV, films, and commercials. She loves acting and becoming new characters. As an actress, Karen observed how when she played different characters, her body would respond in different ways.

Karen had some intense emotional and physical challenges that caused her to seek answers. This led her to discovering ways to transform her fatigue and pain into vibrant energy and chronic pleasure. It led her to fall in love with herself and the world so steadily that nothing can stop her. In addition to acting, Karen now teaches others how to transform their own emotional and physical fatigue and pain into vibrant energy and chronic pleasure.

Karen now lives in chronic pleasure and pure love and has all the energy she needs to do what she wants. She has no stress; nothing is challenging for her now.

Karen has been interviewed by Neale Donald Walsh (Conversations with Neale, Episode 20), Regis and Kathie Lee, Joan Rivers, and has shared the online stage with Arielle Ford, and has been interviewed on countless other TV and radio shows, webinars and telesummits. She was invited to participate in an app with Eckhart Tolle and Thich Nhat Hanh (Insight Timer), and she was invited on an invitation-only expedition to the High Arctic with one hundred world thought leaders to discuss the future and to teach meditation each morning.

Karen loves acting, the local fun dancing, singing yoga class, and doing acrobatics, dance, and many kinds of exercises. She loves eating wonderful organic, unprocessed food that the earth made. She loves being with friends and family. She loves traveling this glorious world. She loves meeting new people. She loves coaching her amazing clients. She loves public speaking.

Karen loves being a benefit and participating in your success.

Her life feels like a magical dream come true.

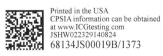